Recent Advances in

Surgery
34

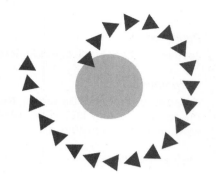

Recent Advances in

Surgery
34

Edited by

Irving Taylor MD ChM FRCS FMedSci FHEA
Professor of Surgery, Vice Dean
UCL Medical School, University College London, UK

Colin D Johnson MChir FRCS
Reader and Consultant Surgeon, University Surgical Unit
Southampton General Hospital, Southampton, UK

JAYPEE BROTHERS MEDICAL PUBLISHERS (P) LTD

New Delhi · Panama City · London

Published by

Jaypee Brothers Medical Publishers (P) Ltd

Corporate Office

4838/24, Ansari Road, Daryaganj, **New Delhi** 110 002, India
Phone: +91-11-43574357, Fax: +91-11-43574314
www.jaypeebrothers.com

Offices in India

- **Ahmedabad**, e-mail: ahmedabad@jaypeebrothers.com
- **Bengaluru**, e-mail: bangalore@jaypeebrothers.com
- **Chennai**, e-mail: chennai@jaypeebrothers.com
- **Delhi**, e-mail: jaypee@jaypeebrothers.com
- **Hyderabad**, e-mail: hyderabad@jaypeebrothers.com
- **Kochi**, e-mail: kochi@jaypeebrothers.com
- **Kolkata**, e-mail: kolkata@jaypeebrothers.com
- **Lucknow**, e-mail: lucknow@jaypeebrothers.com
- **Mumbai**, e-mail: mumbai@jaypeebrothers.com
- **Nagpur**, e-mail: nagpur@jaypeebrothers.com

Overseas Offices

- **Central America Office, Panama City, Panama**, Ph: 001-507-317-0160
  e-mail: cservice@jphmedical.com, Website: www.jphmedical.com
- **Europe Office, UK**, Ph: +44 (0) 2031708910
  e-mail: info@jpmedpub.com

Recent Advances in Surgery 34

© 2011, Jaypee Brothers Medical Publishers

First Edition: **2011**

ISBN 978-93-5025-355-7

Typeset at JPBMP typesetting unit

Printed in India

Contributors

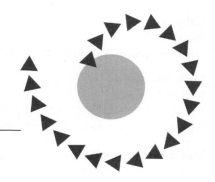

Angeliki Kontoyannis
Surgical Registrar in General Surgery London Deanery
Research Fellow National Institute of Clinical Excellence, UK

Atkin SL
Professor
Head of Academic Endocrinology Diabetes and Metabolism
Hull York Medical School, Hull, UK

Chaturvedi A
Senior Consultant and Head Surgical Oncology
Sahara Hospital, Sahara India Medical Institute Ltd.
Lucknow, India

Colin D Johnson
Reader and Consultant Surgeon
University Surgical Unit
Southampton General Hospital, Southampton, UK

Corrigan MA
Specialist Registrar (General Surgery)
Beaumont Hospital and Royal College of Surgeons in Ireland
Dublin, Ireland

David Jayne
Senior Lecturer in Surgery
John Goligher Colorectal Unit
Leeds General Infirmary, Leeds, UK

Deepak Singh-Ranger
SpR in Surgery
University College London Hospitals NHS Trust
London, UK

Dibor C
Medical Student
University College London, London, UK

Dirk Weimann
Senior Surgeon
Clinic of Visceral and General Surgery
Klinikum Ludwigsburg, Germany

Dominic Simring
Endovascular Fellow
University College London Hospitals NHS Trust
London, UK

Douek M
Reader in Surgery
Department of Research Oncology
King's College London, Guy's Hospital, London, UK

Engledow AH
Consultant Colorectal Surgeon
University College London Hospitals NHS Trust
London, UK

Franks J
Specialist Registrar Breast and General Surgery
Division of Surgery and Interventional Science
University College, London, UK

Hill ADK
Professor of Surgery
Royal College of Surgeons of Ireland, Dublin, Ireland

Jane Cross
Research Fellow
University College London, London, UK

Jonathan A McCullough
Specialist Registrar
University College London Hospitals NHS Trust
London, UK

Khandelwal C
Professor of Surgery
Rama Medical College, Kanpur, India
Former Head, Department of Surgical Gastroenterology
Indira Gandhi Institute of Medical Science, Patna, India
Former Head, Surgical Oncology
Mahavir Cancer Institute, Patna, India

Khandelwal M
Research Fellow
Scunthorpe General Hospital, Cliff Gardens, Scunthorpe, UK

McHugh SM
Research Fellow
Royal College of Surgeons of Ireland, Dublin, Ireland

Mirnezami AH
Somers Cancer Research Building
University of Southampton Cancer Sciences Division
Southampton University Hospital NHS Trust, London, UK

Mirnezami R
Department of Surgery
Hammersmith Hospital, London, UK

Misra S
Professor and Head
Department of Surgical Oncology
CSM Medical University (Previously King George's Medical University),
Lucknow, India

Pearce NW
Consultant Surgeon
Southampton University Hospitals NHS Trust
Southampton, UK

Rachel Hargest
Senior Lecturer and Consultant Surgeon
Academic Department of Surgery
Cardiff University, UK

Richard Cohen
Consultant Colorectal Surgeon
University College London Hospitals NHS Trust
London, UK

Richard JE Skipworth
Department of Surgery
Royal Infirmary of Edinburgh
Edinburgh, UK

Robert Wheeler
Consultant
Pediatric and Neonatal Surgeon
Specialist Clinical Adviser and Hon Senior Lecturer, Clinical Law
Southampton University Hospitals Trust
Southampton, UK

Sathyapalan T
Senior Lecturer
Academic Endocrinology Diabetes and Metabolism
Hull York Medical School, Hull, UK

Simon Paterson-Brown
Consultant Surgeon
Royal Infirmary of Edinburgh, Edinburgh, UK

Sturt NJH
Department of Surgery
University College London Hospitals NHS Trust
London, UK

Taylor I
Professor of Surgery
Vice Dean UCL Medical School
University College London, London, UK

Toby Richards
Senior Lecturer/Consultant Vascular Surgeon
University College London, London, UK

Wakil A
Consultant
Diabetes Endocrinology and Metabolism
Hull Royal Infirmary, Hull, UK

Windsor ACJ
Consultant Colorectal Surgeon
University College London Hospitals NHS Trust
London, UK

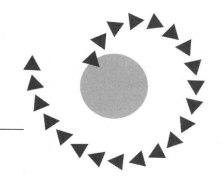

Preface

Each issue of *Recent Advances in Surgery* is designed to provide an up-to-date and comprehensive review of important and topical issues both in surgery in general, as well as in the major subspecialties of general surgery. *Recent Advances in Surgery 34* is no exception.

The general topics covered include the management of the diabetic surgical patient, the issue of patient consent and how guidelines determine surgical practice. The upper gastrointestinal topics covered are gastric outlet obstruction, the relationship between volume and outcome for upper gastrointestinal malignancy, techniques in laparoscopic and open liver resection, and the management of advanced gallbladder cancer. Lower gastrointestinal surgery includes rectal and pelvic prolapse, and the management of an intestinal fistula and the modern management of haemorrhoids.

There is an overview on recent changes in vascular surgery and the management of retroperitoneal sarcoma. Breast surgery topics include the management of the axilla and the role of radiotherapy in breast cancer. As always, we include a comprehensive review of recent randomised trials in surgery.

We hope that each of these important and relevant topics will provide a valuable resource for both surgeons-in-training undertaking professional examinations, and consultant surgeons wishing to keep up-to-date.

Irving Taylor
Colin D Johnson

Contents

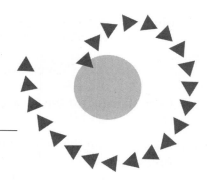

Section One: Surgery in General

1. **Update on the Management of the Surgical Patient with Diabetes**   3
   Sathyapalan T, Wakil A, Atkin SL

2. **How Guidelines Influence Modern Surgical Practise**   20
   Angeliki Kontoyannis, Rachel Hargest

3. **Patient Consent for Surgical Treatment**   34
   Robert Wheeler

Section Two: Upper Gastrointestinal Tract/ Hepato-Pancreatic-Biliary Tract

4. **Gastric Outlet Obstruction in Adults**   47
   Colin D Johnson

5. **Surgery for Advanced Gallbladder Cancer**   57
   Khandelwal M, Khandelwal C

6. **Laparoscopic or Open Liver Resection?**   72
   Mirnezami R, Mirnezami AH, Pearce NW

7. **Volume and Outcome in Upper Gastrointestinal Malignancy**   87
   Richard JE Skipworth, Simon Paterson-Brown

Section Three: Lower Gastrointestinal Tract

8. **Modern Management of an Intestinal Fistula**   109
   Sturt NJH, Windsor ACJ, Engledow AH

9. **Rectal and Pelvic Prolapse**   125
   Dirk Weimann, David Jayne

10. **Modern Surgical Management of Haemorrhoids**   141
Jonathan A McCullough, Deepak Singh-Ranger, Richard Cohen

Section Four: Breast

11. **Radiotherapy for the Breast Surgeon**   159
Dibor C, Douek M

12. **An Update on the Management of the Axilla in
Breast Cancer**   168
Hill ADK, McHugh SM, Corrigan MA

Section Five: Vascular Surgery

13. **Recent Advances in Endovascular Management of Aortic
Aneurysms**   183
Jane Cross, Dominic Simring, Toby Richards

Section Six: Surgical Oncology

14. **Management of Retroperitoneal Sarcoma**   205
Misra S, Chaturvedi A

Section Seven: Clinical Trials

15. **Randomised Clinical Trials and Meta-Analyses
in Surgery 2010**   223
Franks J, Taylor I

Index   243

SECTION ONE

SURGERY IN GENERAL

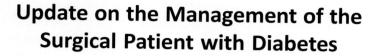

Update on the Management of the Surgical Patient with Diabetes

Sathyapalan T, Wakil A, Atkin SL

INTRODUCTION

Diabetes mellitus is a relatively common condition, affecting approximately 4 to 7 per cent of the Western population. Patients with diabetes have an increased incidence of cardiovascular diseases that coupled with the microvascular complications of the disease which is translated into more surgical interventions. It is estimated that a patient with diabetes has a 50 per cent life time chance of requiring a surgery[1] and the proportion of surgical patients with diabetes is around 20 per cent.[2] Common insulin types and their pharmacokinetics are summarised in **Table 1.1**.

Careful assessment of diabetic patients prior to surgery is required because of their complexity as well as high risk of coronary heart disease which may be relatively asymptomatic compared to the non-diabetic population. Diabetes mellitus is also associated with increased risk of perioperative infections as well as postoperative cardiovascular morbidity and mortality.

Perioperative management of glycaemic control involves a complex interplay of the operative procedure, anaesthesia and additional postoperative factors such as sepsis, disrupted meal schedules, altered nutritional intake, hyperalimentation and emesis that can lead to unstable blood glucose levels. This review will discuss the perioperative management of glycaemia in patients with diabetes as well as management of glycaemia in critically ill surgical patients with diabetes.

PREOPERATIVE EVALUATION

Coronary heart disease is more common in individuals with diabetes. Diabetic patients have an increased risk of silent myocardial ischaemia. Therefore, prior assessment of cardiac risk is essential in diabetic patients before surgery. Other associated conditions, such as hypertension, obesity, chronic kidney disease, cerebro-vascular disease and autonomic neuropathy need to be assessed prior to surgery as these conditions may complicate anaesthesia as well as postoperative care.

TABLE 1.1

Common insulin types and their pharmacokinetics

Insulin type	Onset	Peak effect	Duration of action
Short-acting (e.g. Humilin-S, Actrapid)	30 min	2–4 hr	5–8 hr
Rapid-acting insulin (e.g. Humalog, NovoRapid)	5–15 min	45–75 min	2–4 hr
Intermediate-acting NPH insulin (e.g. Humilin I, Insulatard)	2 hr	6–10 hr	16–24 hr
Long-acting analogue Insulin Glargine	2 hr	No peak	20–24 hr
Long-acting analogue Insulin Detemir	2 hr	No peak	6–24 hr
Premixed short-acting and isophane insulin (e.g. Humilin M3)	30 min	2–8 hr	16–24 hr
Premixed rapid-acting and isophane insulin (e.g. Humalog Mix 25, Novomix 30)	5–15 min	Initial 45–75 min Later 6–8 hr	16–24 hr

All patients are required to have a disease history and careful physical examination, and further evaluation required in selected individuals. Key elements of the initial assessment should include the following:

- Determination of the type of diabetes, since type 1 diabetes patients are at a higher risk of diabetic ketoacidosis
- Long-term complications of diabetes mellitus, both macrovascular and microvascular complications
- Assessment of baseline glycaemic control, including frequency of monitoring, haemoglobin A1C levels (A1C) as well as fasting and mean blood glucose levels
- Assessment of hypoglycaemia including frequency, timing, awareness and severity
- Detailed history of diabetes therapy, including insulin type, dose and timing
- Other pharmacologic therapy, including type of medication, dosing and timing
- Characteristics of surgery, including when a patient should stop eating prior to surgery, type of surgery (major or minor, inpatient or outpatient), timing of the operative procedure and duration of the procedure
- Types of anaesthesia including epidural *versus* general anaesthesia: stress of general anaesthesia impairs glucose control by an increase in counter regulatory hormones in blood including catecholamine, cortisol and glucagon. Volatile anaesthetic agents also inhibit insulin secretion and increase hepatic glucose production. Epidural anaesthesia has minimal effects on glucose homeostasis and insulin resistance. On the other hand, regional anaesthesia carries a risk of

hypotension to patients with autonomic neuropathy and a consequent risk of precipitating a cardiac event in those with ischemic heart disease. Patients with diabetes should be carefully assessed for intubation difficulties since there is an increased incidence of difficult intubation in these patients with a higher incidence of limited joint mobility syndrome or stiff joint syndrome.

PREOPERATIVE LABORATORY INVESTIGATIONS

Basic investigations should include a baseline electrocardiogram (ECG) and assessment of renal function using either serum creatinine (that underestimates renal function) or measurement of creatinine clearance using 24-hour urinary collection. ECG abnormalities are suggestive of previous myocardial infarction and chronic kidney disease which are risk factors for major postoperative cardiac events. Patients with abnormal ECG should be carefully considered for an exercise tolerance test and coronary angiography as the ECG has poor predictive value and 15 to 60 per cent of diabetic patients have asymptomatic coronary artery disease. A resting tachycardia and a lack of variability of RR interval are signs of autonomic neuropathy.

If not previously assessed within the last three months, A1C levels will permit the determination of long term glycaemic control and this is an important element in determining adequacy of current glycaemic management, especially insulin dose in patients. There is also some suggestion that elevated baseline glucose and A1C levels may predict a higher rate of postoperative infections.[3] Further investigations including noninvasive cardiac testing should be considered on an individual basis. Poorly controlled insulin dependent diabetes with high HbA1C levels and impaired pulmonary function tests have been shown to co-exist.[4] Clinically, poor cough decreased response to hypoxia and hypercapnia have been observed, consistent with respiratory function test results in such patients.[5] This indicates the need for pulmonary function assessment in patients with pre-existent respiratory illness coupled with poorly controlled diabetes mellitus.

EFFECT OF SURGERY ON GLYCAEMIC CONTROL

Surgery and general anaesthesia cause a neuro-endocrine stress response with release of counter-regulatory hormones such as cortisol, epinephrine, glucagon and growth hormone as well as inflammatory cytokines such as interleukin-6 and tumour necrosis factor-alpha. These neuro-hormonal changes result in metabolic abnormalities including insulin resistance, decreased peripheral glucose utilisation, impaired insulin secretion, increased lipolysis and protein catabolism, leading to hyperglycaemia and even ketosis in some cases.

The magnitude of counter-regulatory hormone release varies per individual and is influenced by the type of anaesthesia (general anaesthesia is associated with larger metabolic abnormalities as compared to epidural anaesthesia), the extent of the surgery (cardiovascular bypass surgery resulting in significantly higher degree of insulin resistance) and additional postoperative factors such as sepsis, hyperalimentation and steroid use. The hyperglycaemic response to these factors may be attenuated by the lack of caloric intake during and immediately after surgery, making the final glycaemic balance difficult to predict.

The general goals of perioperative management of patients with diabetes include:
- Avoidance of marked hyperglycaemia
- Avoidance of hypoglycaemia
- Maintenance of fluid and electrolyte balance
- Prevention of ketoacidosis.

Uncontrolled diabetes can lead to volume depletion from osmotic diuresis and life-threatening conditions such as diabetic ketoacidosis (DKA) or hyperosmalar hyperglycaemic state (HHS).

Patients with type 1 diabetes mellitus are insulin deficient and are prone to developing diabetic ketoacidosis and insulin should not be withheld at any time. Type 2 diabetes patients are susceptible to developing HHS that may lead to severe volume depletion and neurologic complications and they may develop ketoacidosis in the setting of extreme stress.

Hypoglycaemia is another potentially life-threatening complication of poor perioperative metabolic control. A short time (minutes) of severe hypoglycaemia (serum glucose concentration < 2.2 mmol/l) may induce arrhythmias, other cardiac events or transient cognitive deficits. Hypoglycaemia and subsequent neuroglycopaenia can be difficult to detect intraoperatively in patients having general anesthaetic or sedated patients postoperatively.

GLYCAEMIC TARGETS

Beyond avoidance of marked hyperglycaemia and hypoglycaemia, it is unclear how tight glucose control needs to be perioperatively. There is paucity of controlled trials on the benefits and risks of loose or tight glycaemic control in these patients, with the exception of patients in the intensive care unit or those who have had an acute myocardial infarction. Some studies show that achieving normoglycaemia (4.4–6.1 mmol/l) in cardiac surgery patients or those requiring postoperative surgical intensive care units (ICU) settings may reduce mortality. However, subsequent trials in mixed surgical and medical ICU patients have failed to show a benefit of such intensive control.[6,7] In a multicentre randomised controlled trial (NICE-SUGAR), tight glycaemic control target (4.5–6.0 mmol/l) was associated with a significant increase in severe hypoglycaemia (blood glucose ≤ 2.2 mmol/l) and increased risk of death in the intensively treated group.[8] The vast majority of the patients in these studies were not previously known to have diabetes but developed postoperative hyperglycaemia during the course of their ICU care. A subgroup analysis of two randomised trials assessing tight control in the ICU setting raised the possibility that the apparent benefits of tight control may not extend to patients with known diabetes.[9] Despite some variability in proposed targets, these published guidelines collectively propose the achievement of reasonable normoglycaemia of glucose readings below 10 to 11 mmol/l in these patients. The American Diabetes Association (ADA) has endorsed pre-meal glucose goals of 7.8 mmol/l for general hospitalised patients with random glucose readings less than 10 mmol/l.[10]

Key Points

- We recommend maintaining blood glucose between 7.7 to 10 mmol/l in critically ill patients rather than more stringent target (e.g. 4.4–6.1 mmol/l) or more liberal target (e.g. 10–11.1 mmol/l)
- Hypoglycaemia is potentially a life-threatening complication of poor perioperative metabolic control that may induce arrhythmias, other cardiac events or transient cognitive deficits
- Hypoglycaemia and subsequent neuroglycopaenia can be difficult to detect in sedated patients postoperatively.

EARLY PERIOPERATIVE PHASE

Several strategies exist to maintain target range glucose levels perioperatively but there is no consensus on the optimal strategy. Ideally, all patients with diabetes mellitus should have their surgery in morning as early as possible to minimise the disruption of their management routine whilst being fasted.

Type 2 Diabetes Treated with Diet Alone

Generally, patients with type 2 diabetes managed by diet alone do not require any therapy perioperatively. Stress of surgery may impair glycaemic control requiring pharmacological intervention. Supplemental short-acting insulin may be given as subcutaneous insulin boluses in patients whose glucose levels rise over the desired target. Blood glucose levels should be checked preoperatively and soon after the surgery. Dextrose-free intravenous solutions should be used for hydration if insulin is not given.

Type 2 Diabetes Treated with Oral Hypoglycaemic Agents

Patients with type 2 diabetes who take oral hypoglycaemic drugs should continue their usual oral hypoglycaemic medications until the morning of surgery. On the morning of surgery, they should be advised to leave off their oral hypoglycaemic drugs, although, long-acting sulfonylurea should be discontinued 48 to 72 hours prior to surgery since they increase the risk of hypoglycaemia. However, inadvertent sulphonylurea treatment on the day of surgery should not postpone the procedure if careful blood glucose monitoring with continuous intravenous dextrose is undertaken. Metformin is contraindicated in conditions that increase the risk of renal hypoperfusion, hepatic insufficiency, lactate accumulation and tissue hypoxia. Metformin should be cautiously used in congestive heart failure as patients with heart failure have often co-exiting nephropathy. Thiazolidinediones should be avoided in patients with hepatic insufficiency. Thiazolidinediones may worsen fluid retention leading to peripheral oedema and could precipitate congestive heart failure. Newer agents like DPP-4 inhibitors and GLP-1 analogues could potentially alter GI motility and impact on the postoperative state.

Most patients with good metabolic control on oral agents will not need insulin for short surgical procedures. For patients who develop hyperglycaemia, supplemental short-acting insulin may be administered as subcutaneous boluses, based on frequently measured blood glucose levels that are often obtained on capillary "finger prick" samples. Most oral hypoglycaemic agents can be restarted after surgery when patients resume eating with the exception of metformin, which should be delayed in patients with suspected renal hypoperfusion until adequate renal function is confirmed. Patients who are discharged shortly after an outpatient surgical procedure need to be reminded about potential hyperglycaemia and the importance of seeking medical attention if this develops.

Key Points

- Metformin should not be restarted postoperatively in patients with renal insufficiency, significant hepatic impairment or congestive heart failure
- Sulfonylurea agents stimulate insulin secretion and may cause hypoglycaemia; they should not be restarted until normal eating resumes postoperatively. A step-up approach can be used for patients on high dose sulfonylureas, starting at low doses and adjusting the dose up until the optimal dose is reached
- Thiazolidinediones should not be used if patients develop congestive heart failure or problematic fluid retention, or if there are liver function abnormalities
- DPP-4 inhibitors and GLP-1 analogues could slow down gastrointestinal motility with implications in the postoperative state.

Type 1 or Insulin Treated Type 2 Diabetes

Generally, patients who use insulin can continue with subcutaneous insulin perioperatively (rather than a glucose, potassium, insulin infusion (GKI) or in some instances an insulin infusion alone) for procedures that are not long and complex. If the basal (long-acting) insulin is correctly titrated, it is reasonable to continue the long-acting insulin while the patient is fasting and having intravenous dextrose.

It may be prudent to reduce the night time intermediate-acting insulin on the night prior to surgery to prevent hypoglycaemia, otherwise, the usual basal insulin dose can be administered the night prior to surgery. If the basal insulin is usually given in the morning then the full morning dose is given in those with type 1 diabetes and about 50 to 100 per cent of the morning dose is administered in those with type 2 diabetes.[2] Basal metabolic needs utilise approximately one half of an individual's insulin even in the absence of oral intake, highlighting the need to continue with basal insulin when not eating;[11] it is mandatory in type 1 diabetes to prevent ketoacidosis.

TIMING OF PROCEDURE

Minor and Short Morning Operations

Procedures where breakfast is only likely to be postponed, patients may delay taking their usual morning insulin until after the surgery and before eating.

When short morning procedures are likely to be followed by omitting breakfast and lunch, the insulin dose is based on prior insulin therapy:

- If the patient is taking long-acting insulin glargine at night, then the usual basal dose is given the night prior to surgery
- If the patient is taking a morning insulin dose (short/rapid-acting or short-acting and intermediate), one third to half the total dose is given (total dose = intermediate plus short-acting) in the morning as intermediate insulin alone and short-acting insulin is omitted on the morning of the procedure. Re-start the usual short-acting insulin prior to the first meal. If there is a delay in the first meal or hyperglycaemia ensues, corrective short-acting insulin doses every 4 to 6 hours are given. It is estimated that in insulin sensitive patients, each unit of insulin lowers blood glucose between 2.85 to 5.6 mmol.[6]
- Patients on continuous subcutaneous insulin infusion (insulin pumps) may continue with their usual basal infusion rate
- Start 5 per cent dextrose containing intravenous solution at a rate of 75 to 125 ml/hr to provide 3.75 to 6.25 gm of glucose/hr to avoid the metabolic changes of starvation.[7,11,12]

Long and Complex Procedures for Type 1 or Insulin Treated Type 2 Diabetes

Intravenous insulin is usually required for long and complex procedures (e.g. coronary artery bypass graft, renal transplant or prolonged neurosurgical operations). Studies comparing subcutaneous insulin administration *versus* intravenous infusion have found a marked increase in variability of the glucose concentration when using the subcutaneous route. This variability in plasma insulin has been attributed to the varying degrees of tissue perfusion associated with long and complex procedures. The safety of intravenous insulin infusion in highly monitored settings is established[11,13,14] and their positive effect on non-glycaemic outcomes is well-documented.[15] Insulin infusions are readily titrated because the half-life of intravenous insulin is short (i.e. 4–5 minutes), allowing for more precise glucose control and minimising hypoglycaemia.

Intravenous insulin regimens require close monitoring of blood glucose and electrolytes as well as appropriate interpretation by well-trained staff. Generally, insulin infusions should be started early in the morning prior to surgery to allow time to achieve glycaemic control. There are numerous intravenous insulin infusion algorithms published in the literature with insulin and glucose solutions being infused separately or as a combined glucose insulin potassium (GKI) solution.[11,13] In general, the rate of insulin infusion is between 0.5 to 5 units/hr corresponding to the level of glycaemia.[16] This usually equates to 0.3 units of insulin infused for each gram of glucose with up titration in insulin resistance.[17]

Glucose Insulin Potassium Infusion

In the normal clinical setting, particularly when the patient is not being intensively monitored in a high dependency unit, then the preferred method for providing intravenous insulin is the GKI[18] infusion that is a single solution that includes 500 ml of 10 per cent dextrose, 10 mmol of potassium chloride and 16 units of short-acting insulin, which is usually infused at an initial rate of 100 ml/hr.[17] The solution can be altered depending on the blood glucose measured every two hours by adding or subtracting four units of insulin. Potassium is added to prevent hypokalaemia and is monitored at six hourly intervals and serum potassium should be closely monitored in patients with pre-existing renal disease, especially those who are taking hyperkalaemia-inducing medications such as ACE inhibitors and Spironolactone.

This regimen is fundamentally safe because the insulin and glucose are given together and there is no risk of hypoglycaemia. The disadvantage is that frequent changes of the intravenous solution to increase or decrease the insulin dose may be required according to the two hourly blood glucose results. In patients with type 1 diabetes if the infusion is stopped then these patients can quickly become ketotic.

Separate Insulin and Glucose Intravenous Solutions

With this regimen, dextrose is administered at approximately 5 to 10 gm of glucose/hr, and a separate insulin infusion is given using short-acting insulin. Most type 1 diabetes patients require an infusion at a rate of 1 to 2 units/hr with higher rates in insulin resistant type 2 diabetes. A rough guide to calculate the initial insulin rate from weight can be used (initial rate = $0.02 \times kg^{-1} \times h^{-1}$).[2] The rate can be increased for hyperglycaemia, if there is evidence of insulin resistance or for pre-admission high insulin requirements. On the other hand, the rate will need to be reduced in those with hepatic or renal failure. The initial insulin infusion can be decreased or increased by 0.5 unit/hr to maintain the glucose targets. The short half-life of intravenous insulin means that if the infusion is stopped then rapid hyperglycaemia ensues with potential ketosis. Conversely, too high an infusion rate (compared to the independent dextrose infusion) may cause rapid and profound hypoglycaemia. Therefore, whilst it is more flexible this practice should be restricted to high dependency units.

Key Point

- In patients with well controlled type 2 diabetes preoperative carbohydrate loading has been found to be safe without any risk of postoperative hyperglycaemia or aspiration pneumonia. However, further studies are needed to determine whether the same beneficial effects of this practice on metabolism and surgical outcomes in non-diabetic patients are found in those with diabetes.

LATE POSTOPERATIVE PHASE

Generally, the preoperative diabetes treatment regimen (oral agents or oral agents plus insulin) may be reinstated once the patient is eating well. However, there are a few caveats for certain oral hypoglycaemic agents.

- Metformin therapy should not be re-started in patients with renal insufficiency, significant hepatic impairment or congestive heart failure
- Sulfonylurea therapy stimulates insulin secretion and may cause hypoglycaemia; they should be started only after eating has been well established. A step-up approach can be used for patients who were taking high dose sulfonylureas prior to their admission, starting at low doses and adjusting them until the optimal dose is reached
- Thiazolidinediones should not be used if congestive heart failure, problematic fluid retention or liver function abnormalities develop postoperatively.

Insulin infusions should be continued in patients who do not resume eating postoperatively. Once solid food is tolerated the patient can be switched to subcutaneous insulin and then insulin infusion can be discontinued. Patients, who were taking subcutaneous insulin in the early postoperative phase, before alimentation is restarted, should continue this treatment along with intravenous 10 per cent dextrose to prevent hypoglycaemia.

SUBCUTANEOUS BOLUS INSULIN DOSES

Frequently, small doses of short-acting insulin are often used to correct elevated glucose levels. Subcutaneous insulin boluses, especially when used as the sole method of insulin delivery can be problematic as they result in wide serum glucose fluctuations; small doses of short-acting insulin are often given when hyperglycaemia has resulted. Subcutaneous insulin boluses should never be the sole insulin regimen in type 1 diabetes, because ketosis can occur before significant hyperglycaemia is present. Small doses of short-acting insulin can be given before meals and at bedtime or alternatively, in patients who ate nothing by mouth, every six hours, usually to supplement basal and prandial insulin to maintain near-normoglycaemia. This corrective insulin should be given when glucose levels are more than 8.3 mmol/l and the doses depend upon the degree of insulin sensitivity of the patient. In lean elderly patients with type 1 diabetes or individuals with renal or liver failure are usually considered to be "insulin sensitive", while obesity or treatment with glucocorticoids are usually associated with an insulin resistant state.

SPECIAL CONSIDERATIONS

Glucocorticoid Therapy

Glucocorticoids are used for the treatment of many disorders and are often given in stress, its doses are given perioperatively to prevent adrenal insufficiency. Glucocorticoids can worsen pre-existing diabetes mellitus and may precipitate steroid-induced hyperglycaemia in others. Glucocorticoids increase hepatic glucose production, decrease peripheral glucose utilisation by muscles and influence B cell function. Therefore, glucocorticoids have a post-prandial hyperglycaemic effect on those with diabetes and on those who are predisposed to developing diabetes. Treatment with glucorticoids rarely leads to ketoacidosis or hyperosmolar hyperglycaemic syndrome.[2] To circumvent the delayed efficacy of oral hypoglycaemic agents, insulin is often preferred to control hyperglycaemia in those patients. Patients on a single daily morning dose of steroids develop peak hyperglycaemia 4 to 12 hours later, so the impact on fasting and post-breakfast hyperglycaemia tends to be less. Insulin requirements are often initially underestimated in steroid therapy but glucose control is usually best established with prandial insulin.[2] A variable rate insulin and glucose infusion may be appropriate in patients receiving high dose or variable dose steroids. Oral hypoglycaemic medications can be used when the steroids dose is low and constant; however, insulin is often necessary for those whose glucose levels are elevated (>11 mmol/l).[19] Twice daily intermediate-acting insulin with short-acting insulin are given as an occasional bolus may be needed to achieve glucose control. A two to three fold increase in the total daily insulin dose is frequently needed in patients on high dose steroid therapy.

Hyperalimentation

Total parenteral nutrition (TPN) and nasogastric/enteral feeds are commonly used in patients who are malnourished or severely ill. TPN, especially in those with type 2 diabetes mellitus, will often increase the blood glucose and about 77 per cent will need insulin with an average daily dose of 100 units/day.[20]

A variable rate intravenous insulin infusion can be used when the patient is initiated on TPN.[19] Once a stable infusion rate of TPN is established then the calculated daily requirement of insulin is added directly to the TPN. Subcutaneous insulin boluses of short-acting insulin may be used if insulin infusion is not feasible.

For nasogastric feeds administered continuously over 24 hours, a variable intravenous insulin infusion can be used initially. The total dose administered over 24 hours can be used to calculate the dose for subcutaneous twice daily intermediate-acting insulin, once or twice daily insulin glargine.[2] Subcutaneous corrective dose of short-acting insulin for every four to six hours may be required whilst awaiting for insulin glargine to become effective.[2] Changes in the insulin regimen must precede any changes in nasogastric feeding regimens (i.e. changes from 24 hour infusion to three times daily bolus feeds). Thus, good communication between the surgeon, dietician and the person managing diabetes care is important. For intermittent enteral feeding, one daily isophane insulin can be used in combination with short-acting insulin doses prior to each bolus and calculated according to a pre-meal and two-hours post-prandial capillary blood glucose measurement.[2]

Preoperative Carbohydrate Loading

Postoperative hyperglycaemia due to metabolic stress and insulin resistance is associated with increased morbidity and mortality.[21] In non-diabetic patients, avoiding preoperative fasting substantially reduces postoperative stress and insulin resistance. A preoperative oral carbohydrate load has shown to improve postoperative glycaemic control, most likely by inducing endogenous insulin release before the onset of surgery. This sets the metabolic state of the patient in a fed state rather than in a fasted state at the time of surgery.[22] Metabolic reactions to surgical stress are consequently markedly reduced resulting in a reduced risk for hyperglycaemia during postoperative nutrition, retained lean body mass, improved muscle strength and nitrogen economy. Although, a considerable number of patients going through surgery suffer from diabetes, this patient group has been denied the preoperative carbohydrate loading drink because of fear of slow gastric emptying and impaired glycaemic control. However, in a small cohort of patients with well controlled type 2 diabetes an oral carbohydrate load three hours before anaesthesia induction was shown to be safe without any risk for postoperative hyperglycaemia or aspiration pneumonia.[23] Further studies are needed to determine whether intake of a preoperative carbohydrate drink has similar effects on metabolism and surgical outcomes among patients with diabetes as demonstrated for non-diabetic patients.[23]

Patients Undergoing Coronary Artery Bypass Graft Surgery (CABG)

For coronary artery bypass graft surgery procedures, the insulin requirements may increase up to ten fold, especially after recovery from the hypothermia, necessitating an increase in the initial insulin rate by three to five times.[24] This increase in insulin requirement is related to the technique of CABG which requires large volumes of dextrose solutions to prime and profuse bypass pump, reversal of hypothermia and frequent use of vasopressor agents postoperatively for stabilisation of haemodynamics. It has also been shown that diabetic patients undergoing CABG who had GKI infusion just before the induction of anaesthesia and continued for 12 hours after surgery had a significantly lower incidence of atrial fibrillation, shorter length of stay and at two years, had less recurrent myocardial ischaemia, fewer wound infections and lower mortality compared to intermittent subcutaneous insulin therapy.[25] A reasonable goal of blood glucose below 10 mmol/l is achievable using an intravenous insulin infusion. The rate of this infusion is dependant on the frequently measured blood glucose and the degree of insulin resistance. One suggested formula is:

Rate of insulin infusion = (blood glucose in mmol/l - 3.3) × multiplier.[26]

This multiplier could be 0.02 and increased when steroid therapy is used (e.g. 0.04). An increase of blood glucose above target necessitates an increase of the multiplier by 0.01 while a reduction in the multiplier by the same amount is needed when blood glucose falls below 5.5 mmol/l. A separate intravenous dextrose infusion will need to be used when blood glucose is below 7.7 mmol/l.[27]

Key Point

- For coronary artery bypass procedures, the insulin requirements may increase up to ten fold, especially after recovery from the hypothermia, necessitating an increase in the initial insulin rate by three to five times.

Intensive Insulin Therapy in Critically Ill Surgical Patients

Hyperglycaemia associated with critical illness (also called stress hyperglycaemia or stress diabetes) is a consequence of many factors including increased cortisol, catecholamines, glucagon, growth hormone, gluconeogenesis and glycogenolysis.[28] Insulin resistance may also be a contributing factor, since it has been demonstrated to be increased in more than 80 per cent of critically ill patients.[29] Hyperglycaemia was previously considered an adaptive response essential for survival and was not routinely controlled in ICU.[30] However, more recent evidence from observational studies indicates that uncontrolled hyperglycaemia was associated with poor outcomes and this has prompted efforts to routinely correct and prevent hyperglycaemia in critically ill patients. However, the evidence to date do not prove that hyperglycaemia is the cause of the poor clinical outcomes as hyperglycaemia may simply be marker of severe illness.

Critically, ill medical and surgical patients who are hyperglycaemic have a higher mortality rate than patients who are normoglycaemic.[31] Patients who are hyperglycaemic following trauma have an increased mortality rate, hospital length of stay, ICU length of stay, and incidence of nosocomial infection.[32] Hyperglycaemia is also associated with worse neurologic outcomes and increased intracranial pressure in patients with traumatic brain injury.[33]

A single-centre trial (the Leuven surgical trial) randomly assigned surgical ICU patients to receive intensive insulin therapy (IIT) or conventional blood glucose management.[34] IIT was defined as an insulin infusion targeting blood glucose of 4.4 to 6.1 mmol/l; whereas, the conventional blood glucose management targeted blood glucose of 10 to 11.1 mmol/l. It was found that ICU as well as hospital mortality was significantly lowered in IIT group. IIT also decreased critical illness polymyoneuropathy, acute renal failure, transfusion requirement and blood stream infections, although hypoglycaemia was more frequent in this group.

In contrast, in larger multicentred studies Normoglycaemia in Intensive Care Evaluation Survival Using Glucose Algorithm Regulation (NICE-SUGAR) trial, Volume Substitution and Insulin Therapy in Severe Sepsis (VISEP) trial and the Glucontrol trial showed that there was a significantly increased rate of severe hypoglycaemic as well as increased mortality and morbidity in patients who received IIT compared to those who received conventional glucose control.[8,35,36] Meta-analyses have been performed in an effort to consolidate the data from numerous randomised trials[37,38] comparing ITT to less stringent glycaemic control in mixed medical and surgical ICU patients have shown that those who received ITT had a similar mortality.[37] In summary, mixed populations of critically ill medical and surgical patients increased the incidence of severe hypoglycaemia with either an increase or no effect on mortality when compared to the more permissive blood glucose ranges.

Hypoglycaemia is the most common adverse effect of IIT. Hypoglycaemia can lead to seizures, brain damage, depression and cardiac arrhythmias, and it is an independent risk factor for death[38,39] Based on the above observations, a blood glucose target of 7.7 to 10 mmol/l in critically ill patients, rather than more stringent target (e.g. 4.4–6.1 mmol/l) or a more liberal target (e.g. 10–11.1 mmol/l) is recommended. This range avoids marked hyperglycaemia, while minimizing the risk of both iatrogenic hypoglycaemia and other harms associated with a lower blood glucose target.

CONCLUSIONS

Perioperative management of patients with diabetes is dynamic, being influenced by predictable and sometimes unpredictable events. There are many specific issues that require further investigation, since there is only sparse data in the literature to guide decision-making. Decisions of which regimens to follow and when will depend upon individual patients and the clinician's own judgment and experience.

Key Points for Clinical Practice

- The author's recommendation to maintain the blood glucose levels between 7.7 to 10 mmol/L in critically ill patients rather than a more stringent target (e.g. 4.4–6.1 mmol/l) or a more liberal target (e.g. 10–11.1 mmol/l)
- Hypoglycaemia is potentially a life-threatening complication of poor perioperative metabolic control that may induce arrhythmias, other cardiac events or transient cognitive deficits
- Postoperatively hypoglycaemia and subsequent neuroglycopaenia can be difficult to detect in sedated patients
- Metformin should not be restarted postoperatively in patients with renal insufficiency, significant hepatic impairment or congestive heart failure
- Sulfonylurea agents stimulate insulin secretion and may cause hypoglycaemia; they should not be restarted until normal eating resumes postoperatively. A step-up approach can be used for patients on high dose sulfonylureas, starting at low doses and adjusting the dose until the optimal dose is reached
- Thiazolidinediones should not be used if patients develop congestive heart failure or problematic fluid retention or if there are liver function abnormalities
- Dipeptidyl peptidase-4 (DPP-4) inhibitors and glucagon like peptide-1 (GLP-1) analogues could slow down gastrointestinal motility with implications in the postoperative state
- In patients with well controlled type 2 diabetes preoperative carbohydrate loading has been found to be safe without any risk of postoperative hyperglycaemia or aspiration pneumonia. However, further studies are needed to determine whether the same beneficial effects of this practice on metabolism and surgical outcome in non-diabetic patients are same as those with diabetes
- For coronary artery bypass procedures, the insulin requirements may increase to ten fold, especially after recovery from the hypothermia, necessitating an increase in the initial insulin rate by three to five times.

REFERENCES

1. Root HF. Preoperative medical care of the diabetic patient. Postgrad Med 1966;40(4):439-44.
2. Clement S, Braithwaite SS, Magee MF, et al. Management of diabetes and hyperglycemia in hospitals. Diabetes Care 2004;27(2):553-91.
3. Dronge AS, Perkal MF, Kancir S, et al. Long-term glycemic control and postoperative infectious complications. Arch Surg 2006;141(1):375-80.
4. Ramirez LC, Dal Nogare A, Hsia C, et al. Relationship between diabetes control and pulmonary function in insulin-dependent diabetes mellitus. Am J Med 1991;91:371-6.
5. Sandler M, Bunn AE, Stewart RI. Cross-section study of pulmonary function in patients with insulin-dependent diabetes mellitus. Am Rev Respir Dis 1987;135(1):223-9.
6. American Diabetes Association. Intensive Diabetes Management. 2nd edition. Alexandria VA: ADA;1998.
7. Smiley DD, Umpierrez GE. Perioperative glucose control in the diabetic or nondiabetic patient. South Med J 2006;99:580-9.
8. The NICE-SUGAR Study Investigators, Finfer S, Chittock DR, et al. Intensive versus conventional glucose control in critically ill patients. N Engl J Med 2009;360(13):1283-97.
9. Van den Berghe G, Wilmer A, Milants I, et al. Intensive insulin therapy in mixed medical/surgical intensive care units: Benefit versus harm. Diabetes 2006;55(11):3151-9.
10. Moghissi ES, Korytkowski MT, DiNardo M, et al. American Association of Clinical Endocrinologists and American Diabetes Association consensus statement on inpatient glycemic control. Diabetes Care 2009;32(6):1119-31.
11. Hoogwerf BJ. Perioperative management of diabetes mellitus: How should we act on the limited evidence? Cleve Clin J Med 2006;73 Suppl 1:S95-9
12. Marks JB. Perioperative management of diabetes. Am Fam Physician 2003;67(1):93-100.
13. Van den Berghe G, Wilmer A, Hermans G, et al. Intensive insulin therapy in the medical ICU. N Engl J Med 2006;354(4):449-61.
14. Alberti KG, Gill GV, Elliott MJ. Insulin delivery during surgery in the diabetic patient. Diabetes Care 1982;5 Suppl 1:65-77.
15. Furnary AP, Zerr KJ, Grunkemeier GL, et al. Continuous intravenous insulin infusion reduces the incidence of deep sternal wound infection in diabetic patients after cardiac surgical procedures. Ann Thorac Surg 1999;67(2):352-60.
16. Peters A, Kerner W. Perioperative management of the diabetic patient. Exp Clin Endocrinol Diabetes 1995;103(4):213-8.
17. Jacober SJ, Sowers JR. An update on perioperative management of diabetes. Arch Intern Med 1999;159(20):2405-11.
18. Thomas DJ, Platt HS, Alberti KG. Insulin-dependent diabetes during the perioperative period. An assessment of continuous glucose-insulin-potassium infusion and traditional treatment. Anaesthesia 1984;39(7):629-37.

19. Hirsch IB, Paauw DS. Diabetes management in special situations. Endocrinol Metab Clin North Am 1997;26(3):631-45.

20. Park RH, Hansell DT, Davidson LE, et al. Management of diabetic patients requiring nutritional support. Nutrition 1992;8(5):316-20.

21. Thorell A, Nygren J, Ljungqvist O. Insulin resistance: a marker of surgical stress. Curr Opin Clin Nutr Metab Care 1999;2(1):69-78.

22. Svanfeldt M, Thorell A, Nygren J, et al. Postoperative parenteral nutrition while proactively minimizing insulin resistance. Nutrition 2006;22(5):457-64.

23. Gustafsson UO, Nygren J, Thorell A, et al. Preoperative carbohydrate loading may be used in type 2 diabetes patients. Acta Anaesthesiol Scand 2008;52(7):946-51.

24. Hoogwerf BJ. Perioperative management of diabetes mellitus: striving for metabolic balance. Cleve Clin J Med 1992;59(5):447-9.

25. Lazar HL, Chipkin SR, Fitzgerald CA, et al. Tight glycemic control in diabetic coronary artery bypass graft patients improves perioperative outcomes and decreases recurrent ischemic events. Circulation 2004;109(12):1497-502.

26. Davidson PC, Steed RD, Bode BW. Glucommander: a computer-directed intravenous insulin system shown to be safe, simple, and effective in 120,618 h of operation. Diabetes Care 2005;28(10):2418-23.

27. Shine TS, Uchikado M, Crawford CC, et al. Importance of perioperative blood glucose management in cardiac surgical patients. Asian Cardiovasc Thorac Ann 2007;15(6):534-8.

28. McCowen KC, Malhotra A, Bistrian BR. Stress-induced hyperglycaemia. Crit Care Clin 2001;17(1):107-24.

29. Saberi F, Heyland D, Lam M, et al. Prevalence, incidence, and clinical resolution of insulin resistance in critically ill patients: an observational study. JPEN J Parenter Enteral Nutr 2008;32(3):227-35.

30. Robinson LE, van Soeren MH. Insulin resistance and hyperglycemia in critical illness: role of insulin in glycaemic control. AACN Clin Issues 2004;15(1):45-62.

31. Krinsley JS. Association between hyperglycaemia and increased hospital mortality in a heterogeneous population of critically ill patients. Mayo Clin Proc 2003;78(12):1471-8.

32. Sung J, Bochicchio GV, Joshi M, et al. Admission hyperglycaemia is predictive of outcome in critically ill trauma patients. J Trauma 2005;59(1):80-3.

33. Jeremitsky E, Omert LA, Dunham CM, et al. The impact of hyperglycaemia on patients with severe brain injury. J Trauma 2005;58(1):47-50.

34. van den Berghe G, Wouters P, Weekers F, et al. Intensive insulin therapy in the critically ill patients. N Engl J Med 2001;345(19):1359-67.

35. Brunkhorst FM, Engel C, Bloos F, et al. Intensive insulin therapy and pentastarch resuscitation in severe sepsis. N Engl J Med 2008;358(2):125-39.

36. Preiser JC, Devos P, Ruiz-Santana S, et al. A prospective randomised multi-centre controlled trial on tight glucose control by intensive insulin therapy in adult intensive care units: the Glucontrol study. Intensive Care Med 2009;35(10):1738-48.

37. Griesdale DE, de Souza RJ, van Dam RM, et al. Intensive insulin therapy and mortality among critically ill patients: a meta-analysis including NICE-SUGAR study data. CMAJ 2009;180(8):821-7.

38. Wiener RS, Wiener DC, Larson RJ. Benefits and risks of tight glucose control in critically ill adults: a meta-analysis. JAMA 2008;300(8):933-44.

39. Krinsley JS, Grover A. Severe hypoglycemia in critically ill patients: risk factors and outcomes. Crit Care Med 2007;35(10):2262-7.

How Guidelines Influence Modern Surgical Practise

Angeliki Kontoyannis, Rachel Hargest

INTRODUCTION

A medical guideline is a systematically developed statement to help clinicians and patients with decision-making regarding diagnosis, management, and treatment in specific areas of health care. The purpose is to standardise medical care, to raise quality of care, reduce risk and achieve the best balance between cost and effectiveness.[1]

Guidelines have been in use for thousands of years during the entire history of medicine. In the late 5th century BC, Hippocrates wrote the Hippocratic oath. One of its main principles, "Do no harm" or non-maleficence, is today the cornerstone of medical ethics. Though originally intended to guide the practise of his pupils, the oath still holds relevance today and is taken by most new doctors across the world.[2]

In modern clinical practise, guidelines are gaining an ever-increasing presence. There are many sources of guidelines; governmental agencies, medical professional societies, health providers and patient groups. Opinion on the topic of guidelines differs amongst surgeons. There are those who believe that guidelines are a welcome development that can only bring improvement to clinical practise. On the contrary, others believe that the guidelines are an unnecessary external authority that curbs the autonomy of individual surgeon. They question the validity of the development process and the quality of the body of evidence on which guidelines are often-based. There are also those who see the danger of a guideline becoming the only accepted option particularly in the context of a busy practise or a resource-strapped health provider. Others just feel overwhelmed by the sheer number of guidelines available, finding them often conflicting and confusing. For example, a search for guidelines on the management of heart failure resulted in over 1,000 citations.

The scope of this chapter is to address these points by providing an in depth look at guideline development and appraisal so that surgeons are encouraged to embrace this tool, which can be an invaluable piece of distilled medical information. However, as with everything in surgical practise one needs to learn to use it wisely, with thorough understanding of the risks and benefits, always using judgment and surgical acumen before implementing it.

Guidelines are never mandatory by definition. However, there are situations where, by law, a doctor whose practise deviates from certain guidelines may be faced with legal proceedings.

STATUTORY GUIDELINES (SUBJECT TO LAW)

Guidance Produced by the General Medical Council (GMC)

The purpose of the GMC is to protect, promote and maintain the health and safety of the public by ensuring proper standards in the practise of medicine. The GMC was established under the Medical Act of 1858. Over time a range of new legislation has been introduced that defines their powers and responsibilities. The law gives the GMC four main functions under the Medical Act 1983:

- Keeping an up-to-date register of qualified doctors
- Fostering good medical practise
- Promoting high standards of medical education and training
- Dealing firmly and fairly with doctors whose fitness to practise is in doubt.

In 2010 the GMC merged with the Postgraduate Medical Education Training Board (PMETB) and has a much larger role in medical education and training.

To practise medicine in the UK, all doctors are required by law to be both registered with the GMC and hold a license to practice. Licensed doctors are required to demonstrate to the GMC that they are practising in accordance with the generic standards of practise laid down by them.[3]

Good Medical Practise (2006)[4] is the core guidance which the GMC produces for doctors regarding their fitness to practise. This guidance sets out the principles and values on which good practise and medical professionalism is founded. It covers the following domains:

- Duties of a doctor
- Principles of good clinical care
- Maintaining good clinical care
- Working with colleagues
- Probity
- Relationship with patients
- Teaching, training and appraisal
- Health of the doctor.

Quoting directly from the Good Medical Practise Document 2006 "It is the responsibility of every doctor registered with the GMC to be familiar with Good Medical Practise (2006) and to follow the guidance it contains. IT IS GUIDANCE, NOT A STATUTORY CODE, so every doctor must use their judgement to apply the principles to the various situations they are faced with. Every doctor must be prepared to explain and justify his or her decisions and actions. Serious or persistent failure to follow this guidance will put your registration at risk."[4]

This is therefore a situation where by law a regulatory body has the power to remove a doctor's licence to practise, if the doctor fails to justify appropriately the reasons for deviating from the guidance.

ADVISORY GUIDELINES

Although the production of advisory guidelines does not directly relate to an act of parliament in the same way as the GMC guidelines do, failure of a doctor to comply with advisory guidelines can also lead to dispute with an employer or in case of harm or perceived harm due to negligence in proceedings. It is important to highlight that "a doctor is not guilty of negligence, if he has acted in accordance with a practise accepted as proper by a responsible body of medical men skilled in the relevant art" (Bolam test 1975).[5] Therefore, once again if doctors go against the accepted professional guidance than they should be able to justify their actions appropriately.

There are different bodies that produce advisory guidelines.

1. **Guidance Produced by Government** [e.g. Department of Health (DOH) in England, Welsh Assembly Government, Scottish Parliament]

   These are usually service related guidelines (e.g. referral pathways, referral timelines). They are usually consensus statements that are the result of working groups, where invited specialist(s) have been asked to give their opinion(s) to policy makers. Adherence is often strongly recommended by employers (health providers) or government agencies, and financial incentives or penalties are often used to ensure compliance.

2. **Guidance Produced by Local Health Care Providers** (e.g. health care trusts or local networks)

   These are both service and clinical guidelines. Typical examples are local prophylactic antibiotic prescription guidance, thrombosis prophylaxis guidance or blood transfusion guidance. These may be evidence-based or based on other published guidelines (from national guideline developers or professional bodies such as professional colleges/ associations) with appropriate adaptation to the local community being served. They may also have consensus statements from local committees. These committees are usually made up of relevant specialist staff that volunteer their time to represent their department or specialty on the committee. Internationally there is a recent trend for local hospitals to employ professional guideline developers to oversee their guideline and protocol development (Australia, USA). Adherence is strongly recommended and certain employment contracts include a clause regarding possible legal action (under employment law) against the employee who fails to adhere to local protocols or agreed processes.

3. Guidelines Produced by the National Institute for Health and Clinical Excellence (NICE)

National Institute for Health and Clinical Excellence is an independent body commissioned by the Department of Health to produce guidelines for health care professionals treating patients in the National Health Service (NHS) in England, Wales and Northern Ireland. NICE guidelines are evidence-based recommendations designed to promote good health and prevent ill health. They are developed with transparent processes using the principles of evidence-based medicine. The guidelines address both clinical-effectiveness and cost-effectiveness issues.[6]

The stages of NICE guideline development are as follows:[7]

- The Department of Health asks NICE to produce a guideline on a particular topic (e.g. diagnosis and management of colorectal cancer)
- NICE commissions the appropriate National Collaborating Centre (NCC) to co-ordinate the development of the guideline for use in England, Wales and Northern Ireland. The four National collaborating centres are independent centres responsible for the development of NICE guidelines. Each NCC has a partnership of professional organisations, academic units and patient/care giver organisations. The technical team of professionals working at the NCC who support the guideline development consists of project managers, information specialists, health economists and reviewers. A management board oversees the guideline development work. The board comprises of representatives of relevant professional bodies. The management board monitors the operation of the NCC according to the contract with NICE, reviews the guideline development process and advises on changes to the guideline as negotiated with NICE at the end of the guideline development. The guideline team in the centre for clinical practise at NICE supports and advises the NCC during the development process. The main stages in the process are as follows:
- Agreeing the scope, what the guidelines will cover
- Establishing a Guideline Development Group (GDG) to manage the work. The GDG is composed of relevant health professionals, but also at least two patient/care giver representatives. GDGs usually consist of 12 to 15 people. NICE is not represented on the GDG
- Searching for, appraising and building research evidence
- Accessing and incorporating expert opinion when and if needed
- Developing the recommendations
- Consulting the views of stakeholder organisations on the provisional guidelines. Stakeholder organisations are organisations with an interest in a particular guideline. They register with NICE at the beginning of the process and contribute their views during the consultation period
- At the end of the process, the Guidance Executive at NICE signs off the guideline. The Guidance Executive confirms that the NCC

has developed the guideline in accordance with the terms of the remit from the Secretary of State for Health and the Scope, and by following NICE process and methods. The guideline is then published and distributed to the NHS in England, Wales and Northern Ireland.

There are different types of NICE guidelines, which are elucidated as follows:

- Clinical guidelines cover aspects of the management of a particular disease or condition. The evidence supporting different treatments is examined to assess whether they are effective for patients. The guidelines make recommendations on which treatments should be made available in the NHS in England and Wales, in order to ensure the best care is available to all patients. Clinical guidelines sit alongside, but do not replace the knowledge and skills of experienced health professionals and consider both the clinical effectiveness and also the cost-effectiveness of cancer treatments.
- Service guidance makes recommendations on how NHS services for patients should be organised in England and Wales. Both the anticipated benefits and the resource implications of implementing the recommendations are considered
- Technology appraisal guidance assesses the clinical and cost effectiveness of one or more technologies, such as new drugs, surgical procedures and medical devices
- Interventional Procedures (IP) guidance covers the safety and efficacy of interventional procedures used for diagnosis or treatment
- Public health guidance deals with promoting good health and preventing ill health.

The Scottish Intercollegiate Guidelines Network (SIGN) develops evidence based clinical practise guidelines for the NHS in Scotland. SIGN guidelines are derived from a systematic review of the scientific literature. SIGN guidelines are produced by guideline development group members with support from the SIGN executive according to structured robust methodology.[8,9]

The Guidelines Audit and Implementation Network (GAIN) produce guidelines for the NHS in Northern Ireland. Its role is safety and quality improvement in Health and Social Care Services throughout Northern Ireland by commissioning of regional audit and guidelines as well as by the promotion of good practise through the dissemination of audit results and the publication, and facilitation of implementation of regional guidelines.[10]

4. **Guidelines Produced by International Guideline Developing Bodies**

Since the establishment of NICE in the UK, other countries are also establishing guideline-developing bodies. In the US there is an Agency for Healthcare Research and Quality.[11] In the Netherlands, two bodies, Community-Based Organization (CBO) and National Healthcare Group (NHG) publish specialist and primary care guidelines respectively.[12] In

Germany, the German Agency for Quality in Medicine (ÄZQ) co ordinates a national programme for disease management guidelines.[13] All these organisations are now members of the Guidelines International Network (GIN), an international network of organisations and individuals involved in clinical practise guidelines.[12] GIN is the owner of the International Guideline Library: The largest web-based database of medical guidelines worldwide; and pursue a set of activities aiming at promoting best practise and reducing duplication in the guideline world. GIN also holds annual international conferences. The US and other countries also maintain medical guideline clearing houses. In the US, the National Guideline Clearing House maintains a catalogue of high-quality guidelines published by various organisations (mostly professional physician organisations).

5. **Guidelines Produced by Professional Medical Organisations and Societies (Table 2.1)**

Specialist working groups formed by members of the executive, who have volunteered to sit on the guideline panel, usually produce these guidelines. An alternative is that panel members are self-selected or nominated by their peers. The evidence provided varies with some societies producing very good quality evidence-based guidelines and others producing a higher number of consensus statements particularly when addressing topics where evidence is not available in the literature. A search of the UK-based societies relevant to surgical practise has found that the great majority of professional bodies and societies produce guidelines. However, only one society, i.e. British Society of Gastroenterology (BSG) gives reference to their detailed methodology and uses established, and recognised guideline development tools for their production. This is also the only organisation whose reports have a formal application process for guideline development panel members.

TABLE 2.1

Illustrates that a lot of effort and resources are being placed in guideline development and it highlights the need for surgeons to be able to assess the quality of guidelines and judge their content before applying them to their practise irrespective of the source of their production

Society	Produce guideline Yes (Y); No (N)	Methodology online or in guideline document Yes (Y); No (N)	Quality checklist used (AGREE tool*) Yes (Y); No (N)	Nature of guideline work
Association of Coloproctology of Great Britain and Ireland (ACPGBI)	Y	N	N	Regular guideline production on variety of surgical topics. Clinical and service guidelines

Contd... **25**

Contd...

Society	Produce guideline Yes (Y); No (N)	Methodology online or in guideline document Yes (Y); No (N)	Quality checklist used (AGREE tool*) Yes (Y); No (N)	Nature of guideline work
Association of Surgeons of Great Britain and Ireland (ASGBI)	Y	N	N	Regular guideline production on variety of surgical topics. Clinical and service guidelines
Association of Laparoscopic Surgeons of Great Britain and Ireland (ALSGBI)	Y	N	N	Occasional guidelines on laparoscopic topics
Association of Upper Gastrointestinal Surgeons of Great Britain and Ireland (AUGIS)		N	N	Regular guideline production on variety of surgical topics. Clinical and service guidelines. Also refer to NICE and SIGN
British Association of Aesthetic Plastic Surgeons (BAAPS)	N	NA	NA	
British Association of Day Surgery (BADS)	Y	N	N	Occasional service guidelines. Some clinical
British Association of Otorhinolaryngologists (ENT-UK)	Y	N	N	Occasional guidelines on ENT topics
British Association of Plastic, Reconstructive and Aesthetic Surgeons (BAPRAS)	N	NA	NA	
British Association of Surgical Oncology (BASO) including Association of Breast Surgery(ABS~BASO)	Y	N	N	Several guidelines on the management of various aspects of breast cancer
British Association of Urological Surgeons	Y	N	N	Occasional guidelines on urological topics
British Hernia Society	N	NA	NA	
British Orthopaedic Association	Y	N	N	Regular guidelines on variety of orthopaedic topics

Contd...

Society	Produce guideline Yes (Y); No (N)	Methodology online or in guideline document Yes (Y); No (N)	Quality checklist used (AGREE tool*) Yes (Y); No (N)	Nature of guideline work
British Trauma Society	No access to website for non members	NA	NA	
Royal College of Physicians and Surgeons of Glasgow (RCPSG)	N	N	N	Provide links to SIGN
Royal College of Surgeons of Edinburgh (RCSE)	N	N	N	Provide links to SIGN
Royal College of Surgeons of England (RCS)	Y	N	N	RCS hosts the National Collaborating Centre for Acute Care (NCC-AC) producing NICE guidelines. It also has the Clinical Effectiveness Unit (CEU) producing documents that audit and disseminate best surgical practise
Royal College of Surgeons of Ireland (RCSI)	Y	N	N	First guideline under development on Quality Assurance in Radiology
Society for Cardiothoracic Surgery in Great Britain and Ireland.	No access to website for non members	NA	NA	
The Vascular Society of Great Britain and Ireland	Y	N	N	Occasional production of guidelines on a variety of vascular topics

* www.agreecollaborative.org

ASSESSMENT OF GUIDELINES

In order to assess the quality of a guideline the reader must be aware of the principles of evidence-based medicine and apply a systematic appraisal to the guideline. Detailed guides for assessing the validity of practise guidelines have been developed using rigorous methodology (see www.agreecollaborative.org).

The appraisal of a guideline should begin by identifying the scope and purpose of the guideline. This should be clear and the target users for whom the guideline has been written also need to be clearly identified.[14]

The main guideline document has two distinct components, which are as follows:

- The evidence summary
- The recommendations, a detailed instructions for applying the evidence to a specific population of patient.

When assessing the quality of the evidence summary, it is important to check the following:

- All the relevant evidence has been identified through a thorough search method
- The review is recent enough or updated recently to be valid
- The inclusion and exclusion criteria for data extraction are clearly described
- The evidence has been graded for its validity
- The side-effects or risks of treatments are presented along with the benefits.

When assessing the recommendations it is important to consider whether:

- They have been graded for their validity
- The burden of illness, the guideline refers to, is significant enough in the population to warrant implementation
- The beliefs of the patients or the community are incompatible with the guideline
- The cost of implementation of the guideline is a good allocation of resources for the local community
- There are any insurmountable barriers (geographical, organisational, traditional, authoritarian, legal, or behavioural) to the implementation of the guideline.

Valid guidelines create their evidence components from systematic reviews of all the relevant worldwide literature. The reviews that provide the evidence components for guidelines are "necessity-driven", and synthesise the best available evidence. Therefore, some recommendations may be derived from evidence of high validity and others from evidence that is much more liable to error.[14]

Sources of evidence range from small laboratory studies or case reports to well-designed large clinical studies that have minimised bias to a great extent. Since poor quality evidence can lead to recommendations that are not in patients' best interests; it is essential to know whether a recommendation is strong (we can be confident about the recommendation) or weak (we cannot be confident).[15]

Grading schemes have been used for over 25 years. Since 1970s a growing number of organisations have employed various systems to grade the quality (level) of evidence and the strength of recommendations. Some grading systems are based on study design alone without explicit consideration of other important factors in determining quality of evidence. Some systems are excessively complex.[15]

A commonly used grading system categorizes evidence as follows in Table 2.2.

TABLE 2.2

Scheme for grading evidence and recommendations

Grading of evidence	
Ia	Evidence obtained from meta-analysis of randomised controlled trials
Ib	Evidence obtained from at least one randomised controlled trial
IIa	Evidence obtained from at least one well-designed controlled study without randomisation designed quasi-experimental study
III	Evidence obtained from a well-designed non-experimental descriptive study, such as comparative studies, correlation studies and case studies
IV	Evidence obtained from expert committee reports or opinions or clinical experiences of respected authorities
Grading of recommendations	
A	Evidence categories Ia and Ib
B	Evidence categories IIa, IIb and III
C	Evidence category IV

Unfortunately, different organisations use different systems to grade evidence and recommendations. The same evidence and recommendation could be graded as "II-2, B", "C+, 1", or "strong evidence, strongly recommended" depending on which system is used. This is confusing and impedes effective communication.[15]

The Grading of Recommendations Assessment, Development and Evaluation (GRADE) Working Group began in the year 2000 as an informal collaboration of people with an interest in addressing the shortcomings of present grading systems in health care. The working group has developed a common, sensible and transparent approach to grading quality of evidence and strength of recommendations. Many International Organisations have provided input into the development of the approach and have started using it. The GRADE system is used widely nowadays. The World Health Organisation, the American College of Physicians, the American Thoracic Society, up-to-date (an electronic resource widely used in North America; http://www.uptodate.com), NICE and the Cochrane Collaboration are among the organisations that have adopted GRADE.[16]

GRADE SYSTEM CLASSIFICATION FOR QUALITY OF EVIDENCE[14]

To achieve transparency and simplicity, the GRADE system classifies the quality of evidence in one of four levels:

Quality of Evidence and Definitions

- *High quality*: Further research is very unlikely to change our confidence in the estimate of effect
- *Moderate quality*: Further research is likely to have an important impact on our confidence in the estimate of effect and may change the estimate
- *Low quality*: Further research is very likely to have an important impact on our confidence in the estimate of effect and is likely to change the estimate
- *Very low quality*: Any estimate of effect is very uncertain.

Some of the organisations using the GRADE system have chosen to combine the low and very low categories. Evidence-based on randomised controlled trials begins as high quality evidence, but our confidence in the evidence may decrease because of several reasons, including:

- Study limitations
- Inconsistency of results
- Indirectness of evidence
- Imprecision
- Reporting bias.

Although observational studies (for example, cohort and case-control studies) start with a "low quality" rating, grading upwards may be warranted, if the magnitude of the treatment effect is very large, if there is evidence of a dose-response relation or if all plausible biases would decrease the magnitude of an apparent treatment effect.

GRADE SYSTEM CLASSIFICATION FOR STRENGTH OF RECOMMENDATIONS[14]

For recommendations, the GRADE system offers two grades:
- Strong
- Weak.

When the desirable effects of an intervention, clearly outweigh the undesirable effects or do not, guideline panels offer strong recommendations. On the other hand, when the trade-offs are less certain (either because of low quality evidence or because evidence suggests that desirable and undesirable effects are closely balanced), weak recommendations become mandatory.

Advantages of GRADE over other systems are as follows:[14]
- Developed by a wide representative group of international guideline developers
- Clear separation between quality of evidence and strength of recommendations
- Explicit evaluation of the importance of outcomes of alternative management strategies

- Explicit comprehensive criteria for downgrading and upgrading quality of evidence ratings
- Transparent process of moving from evidence to recommendations
- Explicit acknowledgment of values and preferences
- Clear pragmatic interpretation of strong versus weak recommendations for clinicians, patients, and policy makers
- Useful for systematic reviews and health technology assessments, as well as guidelines (Table 2.3).

TABLE 2.3

Summary for quality assessment of a guideline

- The methodology of the guideline development must be robust and clearly presented
- The search dates, engines, databases must all be clearly presented
- The level of evidence must be clear and presented next to each recommendation made
- GRADE is a new system of grading evidence and guideline developers are advised to use this system
- Any cost analysis should be explicit and the economic evidence on which the model has been based must also be graded and presented clearly.

CONCLUSION

Guidelines are becoming an ever-increasing reality in modern surgical practise. Their purpose is to improve quality of health care provision. With a variety of governmental and medical organisations producing guidelines, it is imperative that the modern surgeon is educated in the principles of evidence-based medicine. This way each guideline is assessed on its own methodology and development process in the setting, is going to be implemented. It is possible that the same body of evidence will produce different guidelines when different guideline developers based on different population or setting. It is always down to the individual surgeon to decide on the individual patient's management. Guidelines aim to assist in this process but never replace the medical acumen and experience of the specialist or the wishes of the patient.

Key Points for Clinical Practice

- Good Medical Practice is the core guidance which is produced by the General Medical Council (GMC) for doctors regarding their fitness to practise
- Advisory guidelines do not directly relate to an act of parliament in the same way as the GMC guidelines do

- Advisory guidelines are produced by the government, local health care providers, National Institute for Health and Clinical Excellence (NICE), international guideline developing bodies and professional medical organisations and societies
- The main guideline document has two distinct components: the evidence summary and the recommendations
- Grading schemes have been used by growing number of organisations. The grading schemes are based on the quality (level) of evidence and the strength of recommendations
- The Grading of Recommendations Assessment, Development and Evaluation (GRADE) Working Group has developed an approach to grading quality of evidence and strength of recommendations
- NICE and the Cochrane Collaboration are among the organisations that have adopted GRADE

REFERENCES

1. Institute of Medicine. Clinical Practice Guidelines: directions for a new program. Washington, DC: National Academy Press 1990.
2. Edelstein L. The Hippocratic oath: text, translation and interpretation. Baltimore: Johns Hopkins University Press 1967; p. 56.
3. General Medical Council (2011) [online]. GMC website. Available from http://www.gmc-uk.org/licencing/index.asp [Accessed 2011].
4. General Medical Council (2011) Good Medical Practice [online]. GMC website. Available from http://www.gmc-uk.org/good_medical_practice/index.asp [Accessed 2011].
5. Jones, M. Medical Negligence. 3rd edition. London: Sweet and Maxwell 2003.
6. National Institute for Health and Clinical Excellence (2011) About NICE [online]. NICE website. Available from http://www.nice.org.uk/aboutnice [Accessed 2011].
7. National Collaborating Centre for Cancer (2011) Developing Cancer Guidelines [online]. NCCC website. Available from http://wales.nhs.uk/sites3/page.cfm?orgid=432 and pid=12489 [Accessed 2011].
8. Scottish Intercollegiate Guidelines Network (2011) About SIGN [online]. SIGN website. Available from http://www.sign.ac.uk/about/index.html [Accessed 2011].
9. Scottish Intercollegiate Guidelines Network (2011) Methodology [online]. SIGN website. Available from http://www.sign.ac.uk/methodology/index.html [Accessed 2011].
10. Guidelines and Audit Implementation Network (2011) Welcome to gain-ni.org. [online]. GAIN website. Available from http://www.gain-ni.org [Accessed 2011].
11. National Guideline Clearinghouse (2011) Public resource for evidence-based clinical practice guidelines [online]. Agency for Healthcare Research and Quality's (AHRQ) website. Available from http://guidelines.gov [Accessed 2011].

12. Guidelines International Network (2011) [online]. Guidelines International Network website. Available from http://g-i-n.net [Accessed 2011].

13. Agency for Quality in Medicine (2011) [online]. Agency for Quality in Medicine (AQuMed/ÄZQ)website. Available from http://aqumed.de [Accessed 2011].

14. Strauss ES, Richardson WS, Glasziou P, Haynes RB. Evidence-Based Medicine: How to practice and teach EBM. 2nd edition. Edinburgh: Elsevier-Churchill Livingstone p. 165-66.

15. Gordon H Guyatt, Andrew D Oxman, Gunn E Vist, et al. GRADE: an emerging consensus on rating quality of evidence and strength of recommendations. *BMJ* 2008;336(7650):924-6.

16. GRADE working group. (2011) [online]. GRADE working group website. Available from *www.gradeworkinggroup.org* [Accessed 2011].

CHAPTER THREE

Patient Consent for Surgical Treatment

Robert Wheeler

INTRODUCTION

Historically, consent before surgery protected the surgeon from the allegation of unwanted touching, battery. Although, the theoretical risk of being accused of battery remains,[1] courts have consistently held that this has a very limited role[2] in health care law; modern legal actions flowing from invalid consent are much more commonly founded upon the premise that a failure to obtain consent falls below the reasonable standard of care that practitioners are expected to provide. The expected standard is covered in detail by national guidance.[3] The past few years have provided legal clarification of the law of consent and some of the issues clarified are now addressed.

IS MORE THAN ONE CONSENT EVER REQUIRED?

The great majority of consensual interventions are lawful; legitimised by a single consent: "consent is the legal flak jacket which protects the doctor from claims by the litigations—the doctor only needs one and as long as he continues to have one he has the legal right to proceed."[4]

This simple formula is deceptive, because it is not always applicable. Requirements for consent differ. Female circumcision is proscribed by statute[5] irrespective of the presence of consent and there are other consensual activities that courts have refused to recognise as lawful. These include making ritualistic razor cuts on a child's face in conformity with Yoruba customs,[6] and impalement of the genitals with fishhooks and nails as part of sadomasochistic practises.[7] Consensual decorative piercing of the genitals is lawful, although whether valid proxy consent could be provided on behalf of an incompetent child for such piercing has not yet been tested in court. Other interventions, such as the non-therapeutic sterilisation of a severely mentally handicapped child, cannot be made lawful simply by parental consent and require the prior sanction of a court.[8] This principle applies equally to the proposed sterilisation of an adult who lacks capacity. What is rarely in doubt is whether more than one person needs to provide consent for the procedure.

This comfortable certainty is undermined by the discovery, within the common law, that judicial scrutiny has identified aspects of paediatric practise where both parents are required to provide consent. A senior judge has enumerated[9] a list of circumstances where in the absence of agreement of all those with parental responsibility; the intervention cannot be authorised without the specific approval of a court. These circumstances include non- therapeutic sterilisation and ritual circumcision.

Although not universally acclaimed as appropriate, ritual male circumcision is regarded by the English courts as lawful, and is insisted on by Islamic and Jewish law.[10]

It might be considered curious to equate the gravity of the decision to circumcise with that of the decision to sterilise. Dame Elizabeth Butler-Sloss did not think so: "The decision to circumcise a child on a ground other than medical necessity is a very important one; the operation is irreversible and should only be carried out where the parents together approve of it or in the absence of parental agreement, where a court decides that the operation is in the best interests of the child.[9]"

In the lower court, where the case was first considered, the judge[11] also concluded that circumcision was 'an irrevocable step in the child's life'. But he noted the paradox that whilst reversible changes in a child's surname are in some situations prohibited by statute, no such statutory protection is provided against an irreversible circumcision occurring without agreement of all those with parental responsibility for the child. The judge mentioned no other reason why non-therapeutic circumcision should be singled out from the array of surgical procedures as requiring dual consent.

The *British Medical Association's* (BMA) definitive document at the time[12] "strongly recommends that either the written consent of both parents or of the person with parental responsibility be obtained for circumcision." The statement appears to employ a double standard, implying that although the decision to circumcise is of such importance as to warrant the signatures of both parents, the unmarried father's consent is of a lesser concern.

The GMC's advice[13] notes the centrality of circumcision to the practise of the Islamic and Jewish faiths and thus by implication, that the decision to circumcise is a major one. In the Standards for Practise, the GMC informs doctors that they must "obtain the permission of both parents whenever possible, but in all cases obtain valid consent, in writing, from a person with parental responsibility..." Acknowledging this professional guidance, the courts in Re J restricted the justification for singling out non-therapeutic circumcision to its irrevocability and the fact that it is a "major" decision, without further expanding on what this might mean.

The disclosure of the benefits, risks and alternative approaches of and to a medical intervention is a crucial component of the process of gaining consent. Almost invariably, disclosure is performed in the context of the medical considerations. For non-therapeutic circumcision, the benefits and alternatives, at first glance, are self-evident. The risks are summarised as meatal stenosis, ulceration, bleeding, infection, recurrent phimosis and of a cosmetic result inconsistent with the aspirations of those requesting the procedure. In this light, describing the decision to consent as a "major" one is hard to understand.

But in a wider context, the complexity of this decision immediately becomes more obvious, as it is both a preliminary step to the incorporation of the child into its family's society and a prerequisite for making any acts of worship valid. Paradoxically, the surgeon pursuing consent for religious circumcision in the United Kingdom is likely to be far less well informed of the significance of these "wider" benefits of the procedure than the parents from whom he or she is seeking consent.

In his evidence to a court for determining whether circumcision was in the best interests of the child of a Muslim mother, a member of the Muslim Council noted that:[14] "Circumcision signifies admission of the individual into his group and fixes his social position, rights and status. If a child is not circumcised during that age, viz 5 to 9 years, it will cause him embarrassment." In relation to the obligatory duty of worship, he further noted: "Lack of circumcision will render the prayer or any act of worship null and void." In this context, the "welfare checklist" provided by the Children Act[15] matters to consider when determining the best interests of the child, rather than resonating with the consequences of deciding against circumcision for a Jewish or Muslim child.

Basing judgement on the checklist, the judge acknowledged the central importance of a child's ability to integrate with his family and faith of his community, and balanced the wide-ranging family consequences of circumcision against those of non-operation.

Some surgeons are anxious about the propriety of circumcising Muslim children lest the child later regrets the performance of the surgery. The judge[16] noted that on the basis of the evidence given on behalf of the Muslim Council, the Muslim religion would permit an upper age limit of puberty for circumcision. Since, it is likely that by this age, a child would be able to demonstrate his competence to make a decision to be circumcised, the possibility of deferring the surgery until the child attains capacity emerges. This approach would be equally applicable in families presenting for non-religious "cultural" reasons. If the cultural belief is predicated the opportunity of reducing the risk of sexually transmitted disease, it could be appropriate to put the choice between surgery and abstinence to the competent child.

Thus, when presented with a child for a non-therapeutic circumcision, the surgeon should make all reasonable efforts to get agreement from both parents. If both parents bring the child to the outpatients, it would be prudent to ask each of them to sign the consent form in advance, signifying their agreement having heard the disclosure. If only one parent accompanies the child, it should be made clear that the procedure can only performed with the additional permission of the other parent, given either in writing or in person. It is inevitable that on occasions of obtaining this second consent may prove to be difficult, due to a wide range of reasons. As to whether the reasons are valid is a matter for clinical judgement. The surgeon's duty of reasonable enquiry must be fulfilled but to the standard of a doctor, rather than that of an inquisitor.

But crucially, if it becomes apparent that the parents are in disagreement over the need for circumcision, the procedure should be deferred and the opinions of the parents should be clarified. Until this is resolved, a surgeon would be unwise to perform the operation, unless with the sanction of a court.

WHAT LEVEL OF OPERATIVE RISK SHOULD BE DISCLOSED?

When describing the risks of a surgery to a patient, there is a common and mistaken supposition that there exists a numeric threshold of improbability beyond which there is no need to disclose.

Where the line should be drawn? Patients facing surgery may be at risk of devastating complications, they have no idea about the existence of such complications. Why should an operation on your spine render you incontinent? Or hernia repairs reduce a man's chance of fathering children? Such risks may seem readily foreseeable to surgeons, but are invisible to patients unschooled in medical science. Nevertheless, it would seem likely that most patients would wish to consider these risks whilst coming to a decision concerning consent.

Nevertheless, doctors are comfortable with ubiquitous numeric thresholds to guide their interventions and depend upon on plasma levels, physiological or radiological measurements to carry a patient across a threshold from non-treatment to treatment.

But the numerical risk of most complications of therapy is usually low and may not be caught by a realistic threshold. Is it right that such a threshold should (inadvertently) conceal relevant matters from the putative patient's consideration?

Courts have briefly explored the notion of a numeric threshold. In 1980, a Canadian court[17] held that a 10 per cent risk should automatically be disclosed when obtaining consent; in this case, to disclose the possibility of a stroke following surgery. This built on the American concept of a material risk where a reasonable person in the patient's position is likely to attach significance to the risk.

Since then, courts have steadily distanced themselves from a numeric threshold. Three years later, an American[18] case determined that a complication rate of 1 in 200 would not equate to a material risk. A "landmark" English consent case[19] held that Mrs Sidaway, who had **37** suffered spinal cord damage after surgery, failed to prove that a prudent patient would regard a less than 1 per cent complication rate as constituting a significant risk.

In 1997, it was held that there was no certainty that an unqualified duty to disclose a risk of around 1 per cent existed, in the context of a family who were not told that permanent neurological damage could flow from cardiac transplantation surgery.[20] An Australian case[21] had held that the failure to warn of 1 in 14,000 risk of blindness following ophthalmic surgery fell below the reasonable standard of care.

From the legal perspective, this was the death knell of the numeric threshold. To disclose all risks of this frequency would be impractical. The court was demanding that "significant" risks should be disclosed, irrespective of the likelihood of occurrence. The UK courts followed this lead in 1995,[22] and holding that failure to disclose the risk of spontaneous vasectomy reversal (1 in 2,300) equated to sub-standard care.

The explicit switch from a quantitative to a qualitative approach came in a maternity case,[23] when a patient lost her baby. She had reluctantly agreed to the deferral of her delivery, in the absence of full disclosure of the possible consequences of doing so. Lord Woolf, giving the leading judgement, held that it was not necessarily inappropriate to fail to disclose a risk in the order of 0.1 to 0.2 per cent; but that the correct standard was to disclose ".... A(ny) significant risk which would affect the judgement of the reasonable patient."

In a subsequent case[24] where it was held that there was a failure to warn parents of the risk of foetal abnormality of a pregnancy that coincided with maternal chickenpox, the threshold of disclosure had to satisfy the patient's determination of a risk albeit insubstantial; the court accepted Lord Woolf's dictum proscribing the use of a numeric threshold.

Legal scholars support this trend, warning against reducing the meaning of "sub-stantial" or "grave" (or "significant") to quantifiable (numeric) risks,[25] since such reduction misses the central point; that only the patient can judge what risk is material to them, irrespective of its frequency of occurrence.

The concept of a numeric threshold for disclosing risk is therefore outdated from the legal point of view. There are no references whatsoever, to a threshold either from the General Medical Council or the Department of Health; other than advice, to give information about all significant adverse outcomes.

The commonest question asked by doctors, when discussing the law of consent, is where to draw the line between matters that must be disclosed and those that require no mention. Invariably, they demand a numeric threshold, and are disappointed when this is not forthcoming. Although, it is understandable that surgeons continue to use this artificial threshold, it is submitted that they should follow the lead of the courts, because a better formula that identifies: What needs to be disclosed has been provided for our use. It is better because it provides an assurance that patients will not be "ambushed" by a serious complication which the doctor could foresee, but of which the patient remained oblivious until it was too late for her to avoid it.

CAN CONSENT BE IMPLIED?

In separate encounters, both the government[26] and a national task force[27] have concluded that it is inappropriate to rely on patients' "implied or 'presumed' consent. Although interventions such as the centralisation of personal data or organ retrieval from dying patients are justified in many circumstances, they cannot be founded on consent unless the consent is valid. This has been reiterated by general practitioners' rejection of any data sharing system in which the consent of the patient is no more than assumed.

Neither presumed nor implied consent are terms that describe a valid form of consent and their use should be abandoned in clinical medicine.

These must be distinguished from a third-term, inferred consent, which denotes the situation where a clinician is assured that all elements of consent are present, thus properly facilitating medical practise.

By asserting that a patient has consented to an intervention, we are referring to the state of the patient's mind. Properly informed, the patient has made a voluntary decision, agreeing to the intervention. Normally, the patient then expresses their state of mind orally or in writing. The caveat that a signature is not necessarily adequate evidence of consent, is in part, based upon the anxiety that the signed form may not be indicative of what the patient truly thinks, i.e. his state of mind. But this expression of consent usually suffices, since there is no practicable alternative.

There are circumstances when it may appear that a person has acquiesced to a situation but it is not possible to conclude that consent has been given. The unaccompanied non-English-speaking parent who brings his child for polio vaccination sits in silence with the child on his knee, holding open the baby's mouth for vaccination. Once inoculated, the child and father leave. A reasonable observer viewing this could conclude that the father acquiesced to the procedure, satisfying the legal test for implied consent.[28]

The father, who has never been vaccinated, now risks contracting polio; infected by the inoculum his child excretes.

The father's "consent" is based on fiction, since consent cannot be provided in the absence of appropriate disclosure. It seems unlikely that he would have consented to this outcome, if informed of his propensity to contract polio as a result of his baby's vaccination.

The observer's conclusion that consent has been provided is incorrect, since it cannot be assumed that the father's action is based upon an informed decision.

Implied consent is a term for a legal device that allows an intervention performed without expressed consent to be recognised as legal. It requires that a reasonable observer would conclude, on the basis of the patient's conduct, there was acquiescence to the intervention. It has the effect of preventing a person subsequently denying that he consented, even though he did not do so. This stops patients who choose not to express their consent and subsequently complaining that they have not consented to the intervention.

The device of implied consent undoubtedly facilitates practise. The GMC recognises that for routine investigations, implied consent suffices.[29] However, it qualifies this, ensuring that the practitioner "is satisfied that the patient understands what is proposed". This describes inferred, not implied consent; where the reasonable observer is satisfied not only that acquiescence has occurred, but also deduces that the patient's state of mind is that of consent. The distinction between implied and inferred is not mere pedantry. The state of a patient's mind, in terms of their attitude to consent, is deduced (inferred)[30] by courts when deciding whether contested consent was valid.

This is completely different from merely relying on a patients conduct to licence an intervention, irrespective of the presence of consent.
Implied consent is an unfortunate term, since it indicates that there is consent, where none may exist. In their review, the Organ Donation Taskforce acknowledged that "presumed consent" is a misnomer and elected to use the term "opt out"[31] when considering the consent systems for organ donation.

However, the widespread false belief that the terms are valid leads some of those who need to legitimise their activity to select implied or presumed consent as the appropriate license.

The Resuscitation Council view implied consent, erroneously, as a defence[32] for unconsented emergency treatment, contrasting with cancer registries' recognition that it is an insufficient legal basis for cancer database registration.[33]

The Information Commissioner uses the term.[34] She "does not accept that implied consent is a lesser form of consent," yet recognises that some situations require expressed consent.

In the field of sharing patient information, her guidance has been variously translated. In the Welsh NHS, implied consent is given "where an individual takes some other action in the knowledge that in doing so he...has incidentally agreed to a particular disclosure of information."[35] Although designed to legitimise the transfer of information that is essential for clinical care, few patients whose information is thus transferred have sufficient knowledge of the process to form a view on their approval. This can hardly be considered as consent. In Scotland, **40** implied consent is accepted even though "explicit consent is best practice,"[36] and should become the norm. This, combined with a warning that the use of implied consent is only acceptable under conditions approaching the threshold of inferred consent, means an abandonment of implied consent, in all but name, by the Scottish Executive when protecting patient confidentiality.

The attraction of using implied consent is that no consent is required. Furness' pithy description[37] of implied consent—"provide an information sheet and invite objections"—is accurate.

"Presumed" and "Implied" consent should be abandoned within medical practice. "Opt out" is preferable; denoting that what is required is patient acquiescence, not consent.

IS THERE A DUTY OF SURGICAL CANDOR?

It is now ubiquitous practise that unexpected perioperative complications are reported through local and national risk-reporting mechanism. But does this "automatic" response correctly reflect a surgeon's duty to be candid with the patient he or she has harmed?

One particular difficulty is where an error has been made that is not immediately obvious to the patient but has caused some tangible harm. There may be a temptation not to disclose. However, truth-telling is a cornerstone of a trusting relationship and trust between individuals is central to civilised life. Since "morality" pertains to character and conduct, and has regard to the distinction between right from wrong, truth-telling seems to be, inescapably, a moral activity.

The families' moral education to their children, the universal duties that adults impose on children to "own up" to misdemeanours reflects this need to ensure that ordinary citizens are honest with each other. It also implies that 'honesty' concerns the disclosure of hidden information, not simply the avoidance of the lie.

The relationship between doctors and their patients is not ordinary. It is described as a fiduciary relationship, emphasising the necessity for mutual trust, confidence and certainty (L fiderer, to trust and fides, faith).

In conclusion, considering the fiduciary relationship between doctors and their patients, and the lack of distinction between a lie and failing to disclose hidden information, there is a moral obligation to disclose.

Within the doctrine of behavioural ethics, the central 'good' elements of human behaviour rest upon honesty, probity and truthfulness. From this perspective, disclosure of error would be considered an ethical obligation.

How should the general public approach disclosure? In reality, this can be done by ignoring the ethical and moral obligations outlined above. The man who owns up to scratching his neighbour's boat whilst it was unattended would be perceived to have done the "right thing", but such behaviour might generate both mild surprise, and congratulations on being "decent". Failure to report the damage would lead to a disconsolate but unsurprised owner, resigned to the fact that "no one ever owns up these days".

On a larger scale, viewing "acknowledging error" on Google reveals a robust avoidance of the obligation. "White House strategists conclude that acknowledging error is not an effective political tactic." Such comments recognise the moral obligation, but honour it in its avoidance.

The general tenet of civil law is that the citizen should look after himself. If A is persistently walking across B's field for a period of years, and A fails to inform B of the trespass, then A will eventually gain a right of way. B should have been more careful with the surveillance of his property and has no "cause of action". This theme continues throughout the law of tort. It is equally applicable in other fields of civil law. Much of the law of contract is predicated on the assumption that we do not "own up" voluntarily. It is for this reason that insurers are forced to insist upon declarations of modification of boats and cars as a contractual obligation, because there is no presumption that the insured will volunteer information that would otherwise increase their premiums. Therefore, there is no evidence of a civil obligation to report an error. However, the GMC[38] advises that doctors should disclose, immediately, any harm caused.

Many NHS Trusts regards failure to report a serious untoward incident to the Trust as a disciplinary offence. However, there is no defined obligation to disclose the information to the patient and one can see a potential conflict of interest on behalf of the Trust when deciding to disclose it or not. However, should your Trust take a similar line, reporting a clinical error that could be construed as serious would seem prudent.

From a moral and ethical point of view, patients should also be told before the Trust, because of the fiduciary relationship a doctor has with the patient.

Failing to disclose to the patient does not appear to create a liability in negligence and even if the failure were admitted as falling below the reasonable standard of care, the claimant would have an uphill struggle in proving causation.

From the professional point of view, given by the GMC guidance, full disclosure is appropriate. In the rare case, where disclosure would cause clinical harm, perhaps psychiatric injury, the doctrine of therapeutic privilege will protect the doctor who correctly applies it and withholds disclosure.

As a clinical decision, disclosure of medical error puts the doctor in an unassailable position. The Trust may wish disclosure had not occurred but will hardly make their displeasure visible. Paradoxically, there is evidence that disclosure of error reinforces rather than diminishes the

relationship between doctor and patient.

Even if the admission leads to litigation, the court is likely to view the voluntary disclosure much more favourably than apparent concealment.

Key Points

- More than one consent is occasionally required, when prescribed by the courts
- The numeric threshold for disclosure is irrelevant: Any significant risk arising from the surgery should be disclosed
- Consent cannot be implied or presumed. Patients are entitled to "opt out" and thus acquiesce, but this is not a species of consent
- There is an obligation to disclose surgical errors, even if they are not immediately obvious to the patient.

REFERENCES

1. Chatterton v Gerson [1981] 1 All ER 257.
2. Montgomery J, Health Care Law, Oxford: Oxford University Press 2003; 228.
3. Department of Health. Reference guide to consent for examination or treatment, 2nd edn, DH; 2009.
4. Re W (a minor) (medical treatment)[1992] 4 All ER 627 per Lord Donaldson.
5. Prohibition of Female Circumcision Act, 1985.
6. R v Adesanya, The Times, 1974;16-17.
7. R v Brown [1993] 2 WLR 556.
8. Re HG (Specific Issue Order: Sterilisation) [1993] 1 FLR 587.
9. Re J (Specific Issue Orders: Child's Religious Upbringing and Circumcision) [2000] 1 FLR 571-7.
10. Law Commission Consultation Papers 1995;139(23):119-20.
11. Re J (Child's Religious Upbringing and Circumcision) [1999] 2 FLR 678.
12. British Medical Association Circumcision of Male Infants: Guidance for Doctors. London: BMA 1996.
13. General Medical Council. (1997). Guidance for doctors who are asked to circumcise male children. Available from http://www.gmc-uk.org/guidance/current/library/guidance_circumcise.asp.
14. Re S (Specific Issue Order: Religion: Circumcision) [2004] EWHC 1282(Fam) 236 @243.
15. Children Act 1989 s1 (3) (a-g).
16. Re S (Specific Issue Order: Religion: Circumcision) [2004] EWHC 1282(Fam) 236 @257.
17. Reibl v Hughes. DLR Canada 1980;14:11.
18. F v R. South Australian Supreme Court 1983;33:189.
19. Sidaway v Board of Governors of the Bethlem Royal Hospital. All England Reports, House of Lords 1985;1:643.
20. Poynter v Hillingdon Health Authority. Butterworths Medical Law Reports 1997;37:192.
21. Rogers v Whittaker. CLR HC Australia 1993;175:479.
22. Newell v Goldenberg. Medical Law Reports 1995;6:371.

23. Pearce v United Bristol Healthcare Trust. Butterworths Medical Law Reports 1999;48:118.

24. Wyatt v Curtis. England and Wales Court of Appeal 2003:1779.

25. Kennedy I, Treat Me Right. Clarendon Press 1991:200.

26. BMA News 20th September, Backtrack on Summary Care Record, 2008.

27. Organ Donation Taskforce. The potential impact of an opt out system for organ donation in the UK. London: DH 2008.

28. Hurwitz B. Negligence in general practice. In: Powers M, Harris N (Eds). Clinical Negligence, 4th edn, Haywards Heath: Tottel Publishing 2008.

29. General Medical Council. Consent: Patients and doctors making decisions together. London: GMC 2008.

30. Grubb A. Principles of Medical Law, 2nd edn, Oxford: Oxford University Press 2004.

31. Organ Donation Taskforce. The potential impact of an opt out system for organ donation in the UK. London: DH 2008.

32. Resuscitation Council (UK). The legal status of those who attempt resuscitation. Available from www.resus.org.uk/pages/legal.htm [Accessed 2000].

33. Eastern Cancer Registry and Information Centre. Frequently asked questions about the cancer registration patient information leaflet. Available from www.ecric.org.uk/patients/Patient_Information_Leaflet_FAQs.pdf [Accessed 2006].

34. Information Commissioners Office. Use and disclosure of health data. Wilmslow, Cheshire: ICO 2002.

35. Wales NHS. Intra NHS Information Sharing. [online] www.wales.nhs.uk. [Accessed January 2011].

36. NHS Scotland. (2003). NHS Code of Practice on Protecting Patient Confidentiality. Scottish Executive. Available from www.confidentiality. scot.nhs.uk/publications.

37. Furness P. Consent to using human tissue. BMJ 2003;327(7418):759-60.

38. General Medical Council. Good Medical Practice. Para 30. London: GMC 2006.

SECTION TWO

UPPER GASTROINTESTINAL TRACT/HEPATO-PANCREATIC-BILIARY TRACT

CHAPTER FOUR

Gastric Outlet Obstruction in Adults

Colin D Johnson

INTRODUCTION

Gastric outlet obstruction (GOO) arises when there is occlusion of the lumen of the gastric antrum, pylorus or duodenum, leading to gastric stasis and vomiting. Typically, the patient becomes alkalotic, as a consequence of loss of gastric acid secretions, without parallel loss of alkaline pancreatic and biliary secretions which enter the duodenum beyond the point of obstruction. Obstruction of the third or fourth parts of the duodenum will lead to copious vomiting with fluid and electrolyte loss, without alkalosis.

Nowadays, the majority of cases of GOO are caused by malignancy of either the gastric antrum or pancreas.[1] Occasionally, duodenal tumours are present with this clinical features. With the well-documented decline in incidence of duodenal ulcer, effective acid suppression with proton pump inhibitors (PPI) and eradication treatment for *Helicobacter pylori*, benign stricture secondary to peptic ulcer is now a rare cause of GOO. Occasionally, chronic pancreatitis leads to duodenal stricture and this may cause confusion in the diagnosis of the pancreatic condition. Intraluminal objects such as gallstones, trichobezoars or foreign bodies are also reported as the causes of GOO. Infantile pyloric stenosis is a separate well-defined condition and hence not considered here.

Metabolic Disturbance

The classical features of GOO are dehydration with hypochloraemic and hypokalaemic alkalosis. Gastric juice contains high concentrations (30–40 mmol/L) of potassium, and chloride, as well as hydrogen ions, which are lost by vomiting in GOO. Hypokalaemia leads to compensatory sodium and H^+ ion loss in the kidney. Correction of these abnormalities requires replacement of electrolytes and fluid volume; the alkalosis will be corrected by normal metabolic generation of acid. In addition to maintenance fluids, the patient should be rehydrated with a solution of 0.9 per cent sodium chloride with added potassium.

Patients with GOO require careful nutritional assessment, because they are at risk of malnutrition due to the gradual reduction in food intake and absorption imposed by the obstruction. Nutritional supplements or parenteral nutrition may be needed before surgical intervention.

MANAGEMENT OF GOO

GOO Caused By Malignancy

About 10 per cent of pancreatic cancers lead to symptomatic duodenal obstruction and require intervention to relieve the symptoms. Cancer of the stomach affects a similar number; cancer of the distal stomach may invade the duodenum or grow exophyticly into the lumen of the gastric antrum. This cancer commonly presents with gastric outlet or duodenal obstruction. Although some of these patients develop symptoms very close to the end of life and are managed by medical therapies only, surgical centres treating pancreatic and gastric cancer can treat at least 10 to 12 cases per year in whom symptoms of duodenal obstruction arise at the time of or shortly after diagnosis. Intervention is required to relieve these distressing symptoms.

These patients are difficult to manage, they are malnourished because of failure to eat and absorb food, they may be dehydrated and sodium depleted from inadequate fluid intake and loss by vomiting. These factors lead to high rates of complications from surgical treatment. Urgent treatment is required not only to reverse these adverse consequences of the disease but also because expected survival is short. Unless duodenal obstruction can be treated with good relief of symptoms and uncomplicated recovery, these patients are unlikely to be offered palliative chemotherapy and will experience poor quality of life.

The management options for malignant duodenal obstruction have changed in last 10 years. Previously, open surgery had reported high morbidity and mortality rates up to 15 per cent.[2] Improvements in perioperative care have helped to reduce mortality rates but open surgery still entails a mean hospital stay of 7 to 10 days. Surgical bypass can be achieved with fewer complications in many centres by laparoscopic or laparoscopic-assisted surgery, which usually leads to more rapid recovery. After laparoscopic surgery postoperative stay is reduced to 2 to 3 days in some reports.[3-5] Therefore, historical data on surgical complication rates can not be used for comparison with other treatments but recent publications on surgical outcomes are few.

Key Point

- Surgical treatment with modern anaesthesia and a laparoscopic approach can deliver good palliation with acceptable low complication and mortality rates.

Antecolic or Retrocolic Anastomosis

There is little hard evidence to guide the surgeon on how best to make the gastrojejunal anastomosis. An antecolic procedure is easy and quick to perform and is usually chosen for a laparoscopic or laparoscopic-assisted procedure. The mobile small bowel is brought in front of the colon and anastomosed to the anterior wall of the stomach. This may be difficult when the omentum is bulky (not often the case when the patient has GOO!) or if the mesentery is short. A theoretical disadvantage is that the stomach may drain less well, particularly when the patient is in bed after operation, because the new stoma is not near the dependent posterior wall and greater curve.

A retrocolic anastomosis is most easily created after delivery of the posterior gastric wall through the mesocolon into the infracolic compartment. After completion, the anastomosis then lies comfortably at the level of the mesocolon. This route may promote earlier gastric drainage but it is less accessible through a small abdominal incision. Retrocolic anastomosis is appropriate when bypass is done in the context of irresectable tumour after trial dissection.

Key Point

- The choice of antecolic or retrocolic anastomosis may be dictated by operative findings.

Open, Laparoscopic or Laparoscopic-Assisted?

For the relief of symptomatic GOO, modern surgical techniques offer less invasive approaches, so that a large upper abdominal incision can be avoided. There is some evidence that this is beneficial for the patient. Guzman, et al.[6] found no difference in outcomes in a retrospective comparison of open and laparoscopic bypass but Navarra, et al.[3] in a non-blinded randomised study (12 patients per group) showed a reduction in mean intra-operative blood loss after laparoscopic gastrojejunostomy. Time to oral solid food intake was longer after open gastrojejunostomy. Two patients after open surgery experienced postoperative delayed gastric empting, whereas no patient experienced such a complication after the laparoscopic approach. In units where advanced laparoscopic skills are available, this approach has been widely adopted.

Significant problems encountered in the purely laparoscopic approach are the difficulty sometimes experienced in the identification of the proximal jejunum close to the duodenojejunal flexure and the need to ensure creation of an adequate anastomosis without angulation of the bowel. Application of a laparoscopic stapler to the small bowel high in the abdomen may be awkward. For these reasons, some surgeons prefer a laparoscopic-assisted approach to identify small bowel and stomach, **49** with creation of a short subcostal incision to deliver the two organs and create a hand-sewn anastomosis. This approach seems to give as rapid recovery as the fully laparoscopic procedure.

Key Point

- Laparoscopic or laparoscopic-assisted surgery promotes rapid postoperative recovery.

Prevention of GOO

In some patients the question of prophylactic duodenal bypass may arise. This is usually the case when a patient undergoes surgery for attempted resection and the tumour is found to be inoperable. If the patient has symptoms of GOO; it is obviously appropriate to do a bypass and relieve the obstruction. In the absence of symptoms, however, the surgeon must weigh the possible advantage of prevention of later symptoms against the potential disadvantage of increased operative complications. Patients with pancreatic and peri-ampullary malignancy may also require hepaticojejunostomy for relief or prevention of obstructive jaundice.

A recent Cochrane review[7] has covered this dilemma. The review found two randomised trials of prophylactic gastrojejunostomy (vs. no procedure) in patients with inoperable pancreatic cancer. In both trials, patients were found to be irresectable during exploratory laparotomy. Most of the patients also underwent biliary-enteric drainage. Overall survival was similar in the two groups (HR 1.02; 95% CI 0.84–1.25), as were perioperative mortality, complications, quality of life and hospital stay (mean difference 0.97 days; 95%CI 0.18–2.12). The proportion of patients who developed late gastric outlet obstruction was significantly lower in the prophylactic gastrojejunostomy group (2/80; 2.5%) compared with 20/72 (28%) when no gastrojejunostomy was done (RR 0.10; 95% CI 0.03–0.37). The operating time was significantly longer in the gastrojejunostomy group compared with no gastrojejunostomy group (mean difference 45.00 minutes; 95% CI 21.39–68.61). The authors of the review concluded that addition of a prophylactic gastrojejunostomy was an appropriate step when a patient scheduled for pancreatic resection was found at surgery to be irresectable.

Another meta-anlaysis[8] came to similar conclusions based on three prospective studies (n = 218 patients) comparing prophylactic gastroenterostomy and biliodigestive anastomosis with no bypass or a biliodigestive anastomosis alone. Gastric outlet obstruction during follow-up was significantly less likely [odds ratio 0·06 (95% confidence interval 0·02–0·21); P < 0·001] in patients who had prophylactic gastroenterostomy. The rates of postoperative delayed gastric emptying were similar in both groups [odds ratio 1·93 (95% 0·57–6·53); P = 0·290], as were morbidity and

mortality rates.

Key Point

- During operation at which a pancreatic head tumour is found to be irresectable, the patient will benefit from a prophylactic gastroenterostomy.

Duodenal Stents

An alternative to surgical bypass is endoluminal stenting. Duodenal stents are self-expanding metal mesh tubes which can be placed in the lumen of the obstructed duodenum to restore the normal food channel. They are placed by endoscopic or radiology-guided delivery systems. Because there is no abdominal incision, hospital stay after the procedure can be short (1–3 days) and general anaesthesia can be avoided. Some series report 50 per cent of cases treated as day cases. Uncontrolled case series[9,10] report impressive results with this approach. Because it is perceived to be less invasive, stenting may be offered to patients deemed too frail for surgery. A systematic review[11] demonstrated that the reported 30-day mortality after stenting was 20 per cent. This review also indicates uncertainty in the choice of these two treatments with differing advantages and disadvantages. Early clinical success and late recurrent symptoms were more often seen with stenting; initial hospital stay, and overall survival were longer with surgical bypass (Table 4.1).

This systematic review[11] found only 2 RCTs, comparing stent to laparoscopic or open surgery containing 27 and 18 patients respectively,[12,13] too small to demonstrate important differences in treatment effect. A further small randomised trial has been reported.[14,15] This recruited 39 patients randomised to endoscopic stent or (usually) open surgery. That trial showed more rapid improvement of eating with duodenal stent but more prolonged improvement after surgery. No difference was seen in median survival (stent 56 days; surgery 78 days). The initial costs were less after stenting (• 4820) than open surgery (• 8315). However, duration of improved symptoms was greater after surgery and the authors calculated a relatively small cost-effectiveness ratio of • 164 per extra day of symptom relief for surgical bypass.

In six comparative studies and 36 series that evaluated either stent placement or GJ there were only five reports of laparoscopic GJ and ten of open surgery, suggesting that there may be an overestimate of the burden of surgical treatment (by inclusion of open surgery data). The major findings are summarised in Table 4.1. The terms "clinical success" and "persisting or recurrent symptoms" are not clearly defined or may vary between reports.

In Jeurnink's systematic review,[11] no differences between stent and surgery were found for technical success, early and late major complications and persisting symptoms. Initial clinical success was higher **51**

TABLE 4.1

Outcomes for duodenal stent and for surgical gastrojejunostomy (GJ) reported in a systematic review.[5]

	Stent (N = 1046)	Lap GJ (N = 297)
Technical success	96%	100%
Clinical success	89%	72%
Early complications	7%	6%
Late complications	18%	17%
Persisting symptoms	8%	9%
Recurrent symptoms	18%	1%
Hospital stay	7d	13d
Mean survival	105d	164d

after stent placement. Technical success and clinical success were not always clearly defined. Recurrent obstructive symptoms requiring repeat intervention were more common after stent placement. Hospital stay was prolonged after surgery compared to stent placement. Mean survival was longer after surgery than stent but this may reflect case selection (stent 105 days, surgery 164 days). Subsequent series support the main findings of this systematic review.[9,10,16,17] We continue to see case series which report a highly selected segment of the patient population, for example those deemed unsuitable for surgery on subjective clinical grounds.[10] There is little published information about the proportion of patients able to return to eating a normal diet, especially after surgery. The clinically relevant endpoint "ability to eat solid food" is often not reported and is usually combined with the ability to eat a soft diet. Experience with stents is that they enable the patient to tolerate a liquid or semi-solid diet but rarely function well with normal food.

A more recent review[18] has identified improved early results from stenting in series reported since 2007: 98 to 100 per cent technical success and 87 to 91 per cent clinical success (improvement of symptoms). Complication rates remain high at 11 to 43 per cent. The authors point out that repeat stenting is often possible when tumour overgrowth leads to stent occlusion. They also note the evidence that long-term stent function is improved, if patients are offered palliative chemotherapy.

A practical point that is rarely considered in the descriptions of duodenal stenting is the need to consider bile duct drainage before placement of the duodenal stent. Endoscopic access to the bile duct is not possible after placement of a duodenal stent. Plastic stents in the bile duct may be occluded by angulation after deployment of the duodenal stent, and should be replaced by a metal stent. If biliary stenting becomes necessary after duodenal stenting, it must be placed by a percutaneous approach.

Key Points

- Duodenal stents can be inserted with minimal morbidity and short hospital stay. However, long-term results are less satisfactory than for surgical bypass
- Laparoscopic or laparoscopic-assisted surgery is the preferred approach for surgical bypass
- If pancreatic cancer is found to be irresectable at operation, gastroenterostomy should be done to prevent later development of GOO.

Benign Peptic Stricture

The role for surgery in the management of benign peptic stricture has greatly diminished. Duodenal ulcer is less common and effective medical treatments have made the complication of "pyloric stenosis" a rarity. With treatment by PPI, ulcers usually heal without circumferential scarring and chronic or recurrent ulceration is now prevented by eradication of H. pylori which is the underlying cause of most ulcer disease.

Experience with PPI treatment of acute ulcers, that were associated with extensive duodenal oedema leading to GOO, was that the ulcer would heal rapidly, the swelling would subside, and the features of GOO would resolve. It is now extremely rare to see a patient who requires intervention for GOO secondary to peptic ulceration.

In cases where scarring has caused stenosis (usually of the cap or first part of the duodenum), balloon dilatation is now the treatment of choice, as this can often restore a functional lumen and avoid an operation. If symptoms recur a pyloroplasty may be required. A longitudinal incision is made from normal tissue either side of the stenosis (usually extending onto the stomach) and this is then closed transversely to create an adequate lumen. Pyloroplasty is a better option than gastroenterostomy unless the duodenal fibrosis is too extensive for a safe suture line. Gastroenterostomy has a greater incidence of delayed gastric emptying postoperatively, and of late stomal ulceration.

Key Point

- Peptic ulceration is now a rare cause of GOO. Balloon dilatation is the preferred treatment if intervention is required.

Chronic Pancreatitis

A subset of patients with chronic pancreatitis presents with symptoms and signs thought to be due to refractory duodenal ulcer. These patients have epigastric pain and because of reduced pancreatic secretion, they may have acid-induced duodenitis. Because of adjacent pancreatic inflammation there is duodenal deformity and even sometimes duodenal obstruction by the fibrosis in the pancreas and peripancreatic tissue. Recognition of this combination of features should avoid inappropriate surgery directed to the duodenum, and should lead to evaluation and treatment by a pancreatic surgeon, who can offer appropriate surgical treatment of the chronic pancreatitis.

Resection of the head of the pancreas will relieve the pain and the GOO. This may be achieved by pancreaticoduodenectomy but a better option is a duodenum-preserving resection as described by Beger or Frey.[19,20] Complete excision of the fibrotic head of the pancreas releases the medial wall of the duodenum and in my experience always relieves symptoms of duodenal obstruction, if these are present preoperatively.

CONCLUSIONS

Gastric outlet obstruction is usually caused by malignancy of the pancreas, stomach or duodenum. If the tumour can be resected, this is the best treatment, but often this is not possible. Palliative bypass surgery using a laparoscopic or laparoscopic-assisted approach gives good long-term results. Patients too frail for surgery may be helped by placement of a duodenal stent.

Key Points For Clinical Practice

- Surgical treatment, with modern anaesthesia and a laparoscopic approach, can deliver good palliation with acceptable low complication and mortality rates
- The choice of antecolic or retrocolic anastomosis may be dictated by operative findings
- Laparoscopic or laparoscopic-assisted surgery promotes rapid postoperative recovery
- During operation at which a pancreatic head tumour is found to be irresectable, the patient will benefit from a prophylactic gastroenterostomy
- Duodenal stents can be inserted with minimal morbidity and short hospital stay. However, long-term results are less satisfactory than for surgical bypass
- Laparoscopic or laparoscopic-assisted surgery is the preferred approach for surgical bypass
- If pancreatic cancer is found to be irresectable at operation, gastroenterostomy should be done to prevent later development of GOO
- Peptic ulceration is now a rare cause of GOO; balloon dilatation is the preferred treatment if intervention is required.

REFERENCES

1. Johnson CD, Ellis H. Gastric outlet obstruction now predicts malignancy. Br J Surg 1990;77(9):1023-4.

2. Navarra G, Musolino C, Venneri A, et al. Palliative antecolic isoperistaltic gastrojejunostomy: a randomized controlled trial comparing open and laparoscopic approaches. Surg Endosc 2006;20(12):1831-4.
3. Watanapa P, Williamson RC. Surgical palliation for pancreatic cancer: developments during the past two decades. Br J Surg 1992;79(1):8-20.
4. Stupart DA, Panieri E, Dent DM. Gastrojejunostomy for gastric outlet obstruction in patients with gastric carcinoma. S Afr J Surg 2006;44(2):52-4.
5. Ghanem AM, Hamade AM, Sheen AJ, et al. Laparoscopic gastric and biliary bypass: a single-center cohort prospective study. J Laparoendosc Adv Surg Tech A 2006;16(1):21-6.
6. Guzman EA, Dagis A, Bening L, et al. Laparoscopic gastrojejunostomy in patients with obstruction of the gastric outlet secondary to advanced malignancies. Am Surg 2009;75(2):129-32.
7. Gurusamy KS, Kumar S, Davidson BR. Prophylactic gastrojejunostomy for unresectable periampullary carcinoma. Cochrane Database Syst Rev 2010;(10):CD008533.
8. Huser N, Michalski CW, Schuster T, et al. Systematic review and meta-analysis of prophylactic gastroenterostomy for unresectable advanced pancreatic cancer. Br J Surg 2009;96(7):711-9.
9. Lowe AS, Beckett CG, Jowett S, et al. Self-expandable metal stent placement for the palliation of malignant gastroduodenal obstruction: experience in a large, single, UK centre. Clin Radiol 2007;62(8):738-44.
10. Jeurnink SM, Van Eijck CH, Steyerberg EW, et al. Stent versus gastrojejunostomy for the palliation of gastric outlet obstruction: a systematic review. BMC Gastroenterol 2007;7:18.
11. Fiori E, Lamazza A, Volpino P, et al. Palliative management of malignant antro-pyloric strictures. Gastroenterostomy vs. endoscopic stenting. A randomized prospective trial. Anticancer Res 2004;24(1):269-71.
12. Mehta S, Hindmarsh A, Cheong E, et al. Prospective randomized trial of laparoscopic gastrojejunostomy versus duodenal stenting for malignant gastric outflow obstruction. Surg Endosc 2006;20(2):239-42.
13. Jeurnink SM, Polinder S, Steyerberg EW, et al. Cost comparison of gastrojejunostomy versus duodenal stent placement for malignant gastric outlet obstruction. J Gastroenterol 2010;45(5):537-43.
14. Jeurnink SM, Steyerberg EW, van Hooft JE, et al. Surgical gastrojejunostomy or endoscopic stent placement for the palliation of malignant gastric outlet obstruction (SUSTENT study): a multicenter randomized trial. Gastrointest Endosc 2010;71(3):490-9.
15. Jeurnink SM, Steyerberg EW, Hof G, et al. Gastrojejunostomy versus stent placement in patients with malignant gastric outlet obstruction: a comparison in 95 patients. J Surg Oncol 2007; 96(5):389-96.
16. Kim JH, Song HY, Shin JH, et al. Metallic stent placement in the palliative treatment of malignant gastroduodenal obstructions: prospective evaluation of results and factors influencing outcome in 213 patients. Gastrointest Endosc 2007;66(2):256-64.
17. Shaw JM, Bornman PC, Krige JE, et al. Self-expanding metal stents as an alternative to surgical bypass for malignant gastric outlet obstruction. Br J Surg 2010;97(6):872-6.

18. Gaidos JK, Draganov PV. Treatment of malignant gastric outlet obstruction with endoscopically placed self-expandable metal stents. World J Gastroenterol 2009;15(35):4365-71.

19. Beger HG, Krautzberger W, Bittner R, et al. Duodenum-preserving resection of the head of the pancreas in patients with severe chronic pancreatitis. Surgery 1985;97(4):467-73.

20. Frey CF, Smith GJ. Description and rationale of a new operation for chronic pancreatitis. Pancreas 1987;2(6):701-7.

CHAPTER FIVE

Surgery for Advanced Gallbladder Cancer

Khandelwal M, Khandelwal C

INTRODUCTION

Gallbladder cancer (GBC) is more prevalent in the Eastern part as compared to the Western part of the world. It is rare in most of Northern Europe and North America. The highest rates are found in northern and eastern part of India, Pakistan, East Asia (Korea and Japan), Eastern Europe and South America (Columbia and Chile). GBC is the most common cancer of the biliary tract worldwide. In areas of high prevalence, it is one of the most common gastrointestinal cancers. GBC is three times more common in females than in males. It is the commonest cause of obstructive jaundice and third commonest cancer in Northern India.[1] In the majority of cases, the outcome of patients with advanced GBC is not good. It has been historically considered as an incurable malignancy.

Often GBC presents in an advanced stage with invasion of the contagious adjacent organs, e.g. liver, duodenum, colon or bile duct. In this review, the authors' have considered GBC as advanced, if the tumour has invaded the serosa (T3) or the regional lymph nodes are enlarged (N1) with any T and disease beyond that i.e. stage II & III (Table 5.1). The aim of this chapter is to provide an overview of the surgical management of advanced GBC.

The current AJCC stage grouping for GBC reflect the clinical treatment status of the diseases, in most cases. Stage I and II are potentially resectable with curative intent. Stage IIA is reserved for large, invasive tumours (resectable), without lymph node metastasis. Lymph node metastasis is now classified as stage IIB. Lymph nodes along the body and tail of pancreas are considered as distant metastasis. Stage III generally indicates locally unresectable disease as a consequence of vascular invasion or involvement of multiple adjacent organs and stage IV represents unresectibility due to distant metastasis.

TABLE 5.1

Upper GI/HPB

T Stage*

Tx: Primary tumour cannot be assessed

T0: No evidence of primary tumour

Tis: Carcinoma in situ

T1: Tumour invades

T1a: Lamina Propria

T1b: Muscle layer

T2: Tumour invades perimuscular connective tissue

T3: Tumour perforates serosa +/- invades the liver and/or other organ or structure, e.g. stomach, duodenum, colon, omentum or extra-hepatic bile duct

T4: Tumour invades portal vein, hepatic artery or multiple extra-hepatic organs or structures

N Stage†

Nx: Regional lymph nodes cannot be assessed

N0: No regional lymph node metastasis

N1: Regional lymph node metastasis.

M Stage

M0: No distant metastasis

M1: Distant metastasis

* The T and N classifications have been simplified in an effort to separate locally invasive tumours into potentially resectable (T3) and unresectable (T4). There is no longer a distinction between T3 and T4 based on the depth of the liver invasion.

† Regional lymph nodes (N1) are classified into two grades; one for standard regional lymphadenectomy (SRL) and the other for extended regional lymphadenectomy (ERL).[2] SRL includes lymph nodes around the cystic duct (12c), pericholedochal (12b), periportal (12p), hilar (12h) and proper hepatic artery (12a). The extent of ERL includes posterosuperior and posteroinferior pancreaticoduodenal (13) along the common hepatic artery (8), coeliac (9) and superior mesenteric (14) nodes.

TNM staging for GBC as per American Joint Committee on Cancer (AJCC)[3] is depicted in Table 5.2.

TABLE 5.2

TNM staging for GBC as per American Joint Committee on Cancer 2010

Stage 0		Tis	N0	M0
Stage I	IA	T1	N0	M0
	IB	T2	N0	M0
Stage II	IIA	T3	N0	M0
	IIB	T 1-3	N1	M0
Stage III		T4	Any N	M0
Stage IV		Any T	Any N	M1

SURGICAL PATHOLOGY

Spread of GBC is mainly of two types: (a) local infiltration and (b) lymphatic spread. The main spread of GBC is loco-regional, with lesions advancing on the hepatic, hepatoduodenal ligament and lymph nodes in addition to invading adjacent organs such as duodenum, stomach, colon, pancreas etc. There is a direct correlation between the T stage and nodal disease, i.e. deeper the invasion of tumour in the gallbladder wall, the more likely that it has spread to the regional nodes.[4,5]

GBC also spreads by the venous route, along perineural tissue and by direct transperitoneal seeding. It usually does not metastasise early. Beyond regional lymph nodes, the most common sites of distant metastasis are the peritoneum and the liver.[3]

ASSESSMENT

In locally advanced GBC, ultrasound has a sensitivity of 85 per cent and the overall accuracy in diagnosis is 80 per cent.[6] High sensitivity is recorded in the area where GBC is common. However, ultrasound is operator dependent and needs a high degree of suspicion. Ultrasound, occasionally added with colour Doppler is the initial test for GBC. It can also assess invasion in the liver or biliary tree.[7] A patient with a suspicion of GBC should undergo a contrast enhanced CT (CECT) scan of the abdomen. CECT is more helpful in demonstrating a mass in the gallbladder or lymph nodes in the hepatoduodenal ligament and peripancreatic region. Endoscopic ultrasound (EUS) is an adjuvant that is helpful for evaluation of the peripancreatic and periportal lymphadenopathy, especially when combined with EUS-directed needle biopsy of the nodes.

Due to the limitation of the spatial and contrast resolution, conventional MRI is not helpful in determining whether the tumour extends into serosa or not. However, now dynamic MRI using a surface coil may provide more useful information. Sometimes the use of magnetic resonance cholangiography (MRCP) or magnetic resonance angiography (MRA) provides additional information particularly in assessing liver or bile duct invasion and vascular involvement in advanced cases (T3/T4). Fluorodeoxyglucose positron emission tomography (FDG-PET) scanning is also used for staging in selected patients where there is suspicion of metastatic disease in spite of US/CT/MRI studies.[8]

Enlarged lymph nodes are visualised by various imaging methods but the presence or absence of metastasis in each node can be difficult to determine. If the imaging tests suggest that the disease is resectable then preoperative biopsy is not required for diagnosis but EUS directed FNAC from a lymph node to stage the disease may be justified in select cases.

Upper GI/HPB

Levels of tumour markers CEA, CA 19-9 and CA 242 may be raised in GBC and can be helpful when the imaging is equivocal. CEA is more specific (93%) but less sensitive (50%). CA 19-9 can also be elevated due to obstructive jaundice, even without underlying malignancy. They are more helpful during follow-up.

Staging laparoscopy should be performed just prior to laparotomy to exclude peritoneal seeding or liver metastasis. It can help in avoiding unnecessary laparotomy in about 33 per cent patients.[9] Laparoscopy combined with laparoscopic ultrasonography is useful in assessing vascular invasion, regional lymphadenopathy and extent of liver invasion, and it should preferably be done before considering radical surgery for GBC in T3/T4 disease.

SURGICAL MANAGEMENT IN ADVANCED CANCER (AJCC STAGE II, III AND IV)

T2 Tumours with Lymph Node Involvement

The incidence of lymph node metastasis in T2 tumour cases is about 33 per cent, ranging from 17 to 61 per cent.[4,10-13] Therefore, these tumours have to be treated with extended cholecystectomy. In extended cholecystectomy, the gallbladder is resected with a wedge of liver with a minimum margin of 2 cm (part of segments IV B and V). En bloc resection of the lymphatics and regional lymph nodes are also done. The extent of lymphadenectomy is more or less standardised.[13] This has led to improvement in 5-year survival from 40–80 per cent.[13]

The survival of patients with gallbladder cancer is affected by depth of primary tumour invasion (pT) and the presence of lymph node metastasis (pN).[5,13] However, precise preoperative staging is difficult in almost 50 per cent cases.[4] So it is important to establish surgical strategies based on information that is available before resection.

Curative resection of the tumour and its loco-regional spread provides the only hope of long-term survival. The extent of resection may range from an extended cholecystectomy with a 2 cm non-anatomic wedge of liver in the gallbladder bed in segments IV B plus V and lymphadenectomy to an extended right hepatectomy and pancreaticoduodenectomy depending upon the location and spread of the tumour.

Earlier, in stage II and III (locally advanced disease without distant metastasis) radical resection was found to have some survival benefit, but it was associated with an 18 per cent mortality.[14] However, with improved technique and postoperative management, mortality has reduced to 5 per cent and at the same time an improved 5-year survival of 35 to 42 per cent has been achieved with radical resection.[6,12,15-17] Safety and efficiency of major liver resection is now well established. Aggressive surgical approach with curative intent for GBC improves survival not only in T1b and T2, but also in T3 and select T4 disease.[18,19]

Key Points

- Unless metastatic, T3 or T4 disease per se is not a contraindication to surgery
- Aggressive resection should be pursued in all patients and attempt should be made to achieve R0 resection, with acceptable mortality and morbidity

T3 Tumours

In most patients, the disease is diagnosed at an advanced stage where curative resection is not possible. Only a highly select sub-group of patients with locally advanced, but non-metastatic, disease may be benefitted from extensive resections including hepatopancreaticoduodenectomy.[20,21] Such radical resection is undertaken if an R0 resection (negative margins and nodal dissection one level past microscopically involved lymph nodes) can be achieved and patient has otherwise good general condition.

Ultrasonography, CECT, EUS, gastroduodenoscopy, laparoscopy should be considered to exclude metastatic disease. Poor general condition or presence of jaundice may also suggest inoperable disease.

Results of radical resections depend on the stage of the disease and experience of the surgeon. Japanese surgeons have shown constantly higher resectability rates and survival. Increasing numbers of radical resections are being attempted with low mortality and morbidity. In the last few decades, the surgical approach has been in favour of radical resections resulting in consistently improved overall and disease free survival.

The extent of liver invasion needs careful assessment. If there is minimal invasion of the liver, wedge resection with 2 cm margins or anatomical resection of the segments IVb and V of the liver is sufficient. For a more extensive invasion into liver, a major hepatectomy may be required, which could mean an extended right hepatectomy. One should tailor the extent of hepatectomy to the degree of liver invasion so as to achieve R0 resection. T3 tumour in gallbladder neck or T4 tumour usually requires major hepatic resection.[22]

Key Point

- In locally advanced disease, major hepatic resection with extended regional lymphadenectomy may be performed. Adding pancreaticoduodenectomy is not recommended by most of the surgeons

By integrating image T status and data from the frozen section of key lymph nodes, an accurate staging and subsequent decision of resection may be possible.

In cases where direct extension of tumour into adjacent organs (duodenum, stomach, or colon) is suspected, an en bloc resection should be performed as it can be difficult to distinguish inflammation from invasion.

Lymph node evaluation is a critical component of radical surgery for GBC.[23] Liang, et al demonstrated lymph node metastasis in 58 per cent cases with T3 tumour.[12] Patients with N1 disease (stage III) achieve long-term survival with radical resection if the positive nodes are confined to the hepatoduodenal ligament. Positive nodes in more distant groups are associated with poor outcomes. The risk of positive regional lymph nodes in patients with image T3 or T4 disease can be estimated in individual cases by preoperatively sampling the key nodes by EUS and frozen section. Overall, the probability of lymph node metastasis in patients with image T3 or T4 disease is as high as 64 per cent.[11] However, the risk of lymphatic spread is minimal if N12b, N12c and N13a are negative for cancer.[4]

Extended regional lymphadenectomy with or without major liver resection is occasionally indicated in patients with more advanced disease. Enlarged nodes behind the duodenum pose a surgical challenge. While smaller non-infiltrative nodes can be dissected well by kocherisation, larger and infiltrative nodes cannot be satisfactorily removed without the addition of pancreaticoduodenectomy. The presence of peripancreatic (head only) lymph node disease is not an absolute contraindication. Shirai Y, et al recommended combined pancreaticoduodenectomy and hepatectomy in locally advanced gallbladder cancer but only if a potentially curative resection is feasible.[24] However, there is no survival advantage to such radical procedures.[4,12]

Many authors from Japan have attempted pancreaticoduodenectomy combined with hepatic resection, but postoperative complications are high.[20,21]

If the N13a node (peripancreatic posterosuperior node) is negative for cancer, the chances of involvement of coeliac and superior mesenteric nodes is less than 20 per cent and extended regional lymphadenectomy to clear any local extension is worth a try in such cases.[4] If necessary, resection of an involved adjacent organ is also justified. In duodenal infiltration, R0 resection can be performed with either a duodenal sleeve resection or distal gastrectomy with resection of the first part of duodenum. There is no need to perform pancreatoduodenecomy.[25] Patients with N8a, N8b, N13 or greater disease do not survive long and are beyond the reach of curative resection. Evidence of such lymph node disease on preoperative imaging precludes curative resection.

Liver resection with concomitant pancreaticoduodenectomy becomes a formidable operation. Addition of pancreaticoduodenectomy to major liver resection needs careful judgement between the high morbidity and mortality associated with it and the doubtful survival benefit in presence of gross regional lymphadenopathy.

> **Key Points**
>
> - Routine resection of bile duct in extended cholecystectomy is not recommended
> - If the tumour has invaded organs like duodenum, stomach or colon then limited resection (wedge/sleeve) should be considered instead of formal organ resection

T4 Tumours

Once tumour has invaded portal vein, hepatic artery or multiple organs/structures, it often becomes unresectable. Even in cases where extensive resections are performed, they are rarely, if ever, curative. As a result, palliative therapies are often recommended rather than radical surgery at this stage.

Overall lymph node positivity is very high (85%) in T4 tumour.[11,12] Extended regional lymphadenectomy (ERL) should be performed in patients with stage III disease without distant metastases, if the primary lesions can be dissected radically.[2,12]

Aggressive surgery for bulky disease has been shown to prolong survival and improve quality of life[14,24] but multi-organ resection (duodenum/colon) can only be justified if R0 resection can be achieved and the patient is in a good general health.[26] Only sleeve or partial resection of the involved organ is advisable.[25]

Where R0 cannot be achieved safely, patient should be treated non-operatively with a palliative intent. There is no role of cytoreduction in GBC.

> **Key Points**
>
> - Once porta hepatis has been involved and patient presents with jaundice, curative resection is unlikely
> - Planned cytoreduction or debulking surgery should not be done.

Consideration of Extra Hepatic Bile Duct Excision

Bile duct resection simply to facilitate lymph node dissection should be avoided. Routine resection of the bile duct is not advisable unless it is involved directly by primary tumour or by a pericholedochal node.[27,28] No survival benefit was found in T2 disease by adding biliary excision over radical resection without bile duct excision.[4,17]

After removing the gallbladder, the cystic duct margin should be inspected and subjected to frozen section, especially if the primary tumour is located in the neck of the gallbladder. If the cystic duct margin is close to or positive for tumour then there should be no hesitation in resecting the bile duct and performing a hepaticojejunostomy. Mirizzi syndrome, papillary tumour or choledochal cyst are also indications for bile duct excision.

Obstructive jaundice in GBC is an ominous sign. In majority, jaundice is produced by invasion of the bile duct by primary tumour or by pressure of metastatic nodes. Rarely choledocholithiasis associated with GBC may be the cause of jaundice.

Together with invasion to adjacent organs, bile duct invasion has been considered as incurable by surgery.[6] In Memorial Sloan-Kettering Cancer Center, USA, 34 per cent of GBC patients presented with jaundice and only 7 per cent of jaundiced patients had resectable disease.[6]

Key Points

- In incidental GBC (beyond T1a) with non-metastatic disease, completion extended cholecystectomy should be done, with an aim to achieve R0 clearance. A delay per se, is not a contraindication to re-operation.
- Palliative surgery for bowel obstruction or jaundice should only be undertaken if endoscopic or other less invasive procedures fail or expertise is not available.

Management of GBC: Post Cholecystectomy

Many patients are referred to a tertiary centre after cholecystectomy (open or laparoscopic) with a histopathological report of GBC. In developing countries, post cholecystectomy patients also occasionally present with a gallbladder fossa mass without a histopathological report. All such cases should be worked up properly including operative details of cholecystectomy. If there was an intraoperative bile leak or the whole gallbladder has not been removed as a single specimen; the role of re-operation decreases. Review of histopathology, T stage, CT Scan and diagnostic laparoscopy are advisable before planning a re-operation. This re-operation or second look operation for resection is better known as completion extended cholecystectomy. This means resection of gallbladder fossa (anatomical segment IVb and V or non-anatomical 2 cm wedge of liver) with standard regional lymphadenectomy. Resection of the biliary duct is not routine and has been discussed separately.[14,16,17]

Revision surgery leads to improvement in survival for tumours that are T2 disease or higher.[19] In re-operative cases for T2 lesions, patients should be cautioned about the high possibility of not finding any residual disease in the resected specimen. In a review of ten years of re-resection, residual tumour was found in all T3 tumours, but no residual hepatic disease was found in T2 tumours; overall 55 per cent of those undergoing re-resection had residual disease.[29] Some survival benefit has been reported in select T3 tumours.[16]

Some surgeons recommend port site removal at reoperation for GBC, however, the exact course of involvement of the port sites may not be identifiable and the benefit of routine port site resections is uncertain. Port site metastases are a marker for a greater likelihood of subsequent peritoneal disease.[30]

A second look should always be offered in selected cases as 5-year survival improves by completion extended cholecystectomy.[16,17,31]

PALLIATIVE SURGERY IN ADVANCED GALLBLADDER CANCER

By definition, a palliative procedure is one which is carried out to reduce the severity or relieve a symptom so as to improve the quality of life. Symptomatic patients should be palliated by minimal invasive procedures preferably by non-surgical methods.

The main presenting symptoms are pain, vomiting, jaundice, abdominal distension and pruritus. These may be manifestations of gastric/duodenal or biliary obstruction. Though palliative resection has been considered in the past; an aggressive surgical approach for palliation is not recommended.

However, once laparotomy has commenced, according to authors' experience, a safe palliative cholecystectomy (without going through the plane of macroscopic tumour) can be done, as it helps in reducing pain and infection. If the tumour is unresectable, palliation for biliary or duodenal obstruction is indicated only if the patient is symptomatic.

Palliation of Jaundice

Obstructive jaundice can be palliated with biliary stenting by endoscopic or trans-hepatic means. If it fails or facilities and expertise are not available then surgical biliary bypass may be considered to relieve intractable pruritus. As the obstruction is almost always at or near the biliary confluence, a segment III bypass should be performed. Intrahepatic segment III hepaticojejunostomy gives good result with a success rate of 87 per cent.[32] Anastomosis at the porta is neither feasible nor desirable in such situations. Occasionally there may be an obstruction of the lower end of the bile duct due to compression by retropancreatic lymph nodes and in such cases common hepatic duct/bile duct can be used for bypass if non-invasive methods have failed.

Surgical Palliation for Bowel Obstruction

The commonest site of bowel obstruction is extrinsic compression of the first part of duodenum by the tumour. Malignant gastroparesis should be excluded. Endoscopic stenting or percutaneous feeding tube insertion should be the first choice. If a gastrojejunostomy is needed, it should be done from the anterior wall of the stomach so that the anastomosis is not obstructed early from retroperitoneal lymphadenopathy. For hepatic flexure colonic obstruction, an ileo-transverse anastomosis can be done. If resection of the involved organ is planned, it may range from a wedge/sleeve resection of the duodenum, stomach or colon to a more radical resection depending on the area of invasion.

Palliative cholecystectomy with an aim of reducing tumour burden so that chemotherapy can be more effective is not recommended. Performing a planned R2 resection for GBC is unjustified as the patient derives no benefit and is subjected to unnecessary surgery with its associated morbidity and potential mortality.

CHEMORADIATION THERAPY

5-Fluorouracil (5-FU) based chemotherapy had been the mainstay of adjuvant regimens historically. Subsequently, Gemcitabine alone or in combination has been used. There are no data to support the use of adjuvant therapy in node negative GBC. Node negative stage (I and IIA) does not show any improvement in survival by adding adjuvant therapy.[33-35]

Lymph node positive stages (T2N1 or T3N1) showed an increase in disease free survival after adjuvant therapy. Adjuvant chemoradiation therapy has been recommended for lymph node positive T2/T3/T4 GBC following surgical resection.[12,36]

> **Key Point**
>
> - Adjuvant chemoradiation is recommended in GBC only for lymph node positive or residual disease following surgical resection. Combination chemotherapy is effective in locally advanced or metastatic disease

In a situation where curative resection is not possible, radiotherapy with or without chemotherapy has been tried but with only little impact on survival.[37] However, recently a phase III clinical trial results have shown that as compared to Gemcitabine alone, the combination of Cisplatin and Gemcitabine has resulted in an improved overall survival of patients with locally advanced or metastatic GBC.[38] Gemcitabine based chemotherapy has also been used as neo-adjuvant therapy. After down-staging the authors have operated on a few such cases and it was possible to achieve R0 resections in select cases. Image guided radiation therapy (IGRT) and intensity modulated radiation therapy (IMRT) are also being used increasingly.

PROGNOSIS

Tumour size (T) and nodal disease (N) are important prognostic factors. Increased surgical experience with safe and standardized techniques of hepatic resection has resulted in a progressive decline in morbidity and mortality associated with surgery for GBC.[39] Actuarial 5-year survival of 83 per cent for stage II disease and 63 per cent for stage III have been reported.[15] In incidental GBC, significant survival benefit of completion extended cholecystectomy is well documented for early GBC (T1 and T2). Even in T3 tumours, some prolongation of survival has been reported in selected cases following completion extended cholecystectomy.[16]

The number of positive nodes is an important prognostic factor. A 5-year survival of 77 per cent has been documented in patients without nodal involvement.[11] Five-year survival rates of 33 per cent for patients with a single node metastasis and 0 per cent for patients with 2 or more lymph nodes involved has been reported.[11] Patients with advanced GBC are expected to survive long if only one of hepatic invasion, hepatoduodenal ligament invasion or lymph node metastasis is positive.[40]

The overall prognosis in GBC remains grim with 5-year survival of less than 5 to 15 per cent.[35] Extended resection in selected cases of advanced GBC can increase the 5-year survival.[41] Stage II patients can expect a 5-year survival of 30 to 40 per cent but in stage IV disease survival is 0 per cent. Exploratory laparotomy which reveals inoperable disease has a negative impact on survival.[42] Adjuvant chemoradiation therapy is associated with improved survival in patients with loco-regional disease, especially in patients who underwent a non-curative resection.[12]

SUMMARY

Every attempt should be made to resect the tumour and to achieve R0 clearance. An aggressive resection policy should be pursued in all patients as it gives the only chance of long term survival. R0 resection clearly improves survival. Surgery offers the only possibility of cure. Improvement in mortality and morbidity rates following major liver resections has led to more radical surgery in locally advanced cases. Over the years, Japan and now Europe and North America have shown improvements in 5-year survival by aggressive surgery in locally advanced (stage II and III) GBC.

Preoperative assessment for achieving R0 resection is crucial, whether it is for a primary extended cholecystectomy or a completion extended cholecystectomy. A delay between simple cholecystectomy and subsequent completion extended cholecystectomy does not worsen the prognosis. The magnitude of surgery will depend on the local spread of the disease but wedge resection (Segments IVB and V of liver) of the gallbladder fossa and SRL is the minimum (for disease beyond T1a) and may extend to extended right hepatectomy and ERL.

Limited resection of involved organs (duodenum, stomach, colon) may also be required to achieve R0 resection but adding pancreatico-duodenectomy is not favoured by majority of the surgeons. Routine excision of extra-hepatic bile ducts is not recommended but if required to achieve R0 resection, one should not hesitate.

Once the porta hepatis has been involved and jaundice has manifested, the chances of cure are less likely and the decision of resection, if at all, should be taken carefully. Debulking or cytoreduction surgery has no role.

Adjuvant chemoradiation is recommended for lymph node positive T2/T3/T4 disease following surgical resection. Node negative GBC doesn't benefit from adjuvant therapy. Cisplatin and Gemcitabine combination improves survival in locally advanced or metastatic GBC.

Key Points for Clinical Practice

- Unless metastatic, T3 or T4 disease per se is not a contraindication to surgery.
- Aggressive resection should be pursued in all patients and attempt should be made to achieve R0 resection, with acceptable mortality and morbidity.
- In locally advanced disease, major hepatic resection with extended regional lymphadenectomy may be performed. Adding pancreaticoduodenectomy is not recommended by most of the surgeons.
- Routine resection of bile duct, in extended cholecystectomy is not recommended.
- If the tumour has invaded organs like duodenum, stomach or colon then limited resection (wedge/sleeve) should be considered instead of formal organ resection.
- Once porta hepatis has been involved and patient presents with jaundice, curative resection is unlikely.
- Planned cytoreduction or debulking surgery should not be done.
- In incidental GBC (beyond T1a) with non-metastatic disease, completion extended cholecystectomy should be done, with an aim to achieve R0 clearance. A delay per se, is not a contraindication to re-operation.
- Palliative surgery for bowel obstruction or jaundice should only be undertaken if endoscopic or other less invasive procedures fail or expertise is not available.
- Adjuvant chemoradiation is recommended in GBC only for lymph node positive or residual disease following surgical resection. Combination chemotherapy is effective in locally advanced or metastatic disease.

REFERENCES

1. Shukla VK, Khandelwal C, Roy SK, et al. Primary carcinoma of the gall bladder: a review of a 16-year period at the University Hospital. J Surg Oncol. 1985;28(1):32-5.

2. Wang JD, Liu YB, Quan ZW, et al. Role of regional lymphadenectomy in different stage of gallbladder carcinoma. Hepatogastroenterology. 2009;56(91-92):593-6.

3. Edge SB, Compton CC. The American Joint Committee on Cancer: the 7th edition of the AJCC cancer staging manual and the future of TNM. Ann Surg Oncol. 2010;17(6):1471-4.

4. Kokudo N, Makuuchi M, Natori T, et al. Strategies for surgical treatment of gallbladder carcinoma based on information available before resection. Arch Surg. 2003;138(7):741-50.

5. Kondo S, Nimura Y, Hayakawa N, et al. Regional and para-aortic lymphadenectomy in radical surgery for advanced gallbladder carcinoma. Br J Surg. 2000;87(4):418-22.

6. Hawkins WG, DeMatteo RP, Jarnagin WR, et al. Jaundice predicts advanced disease and early mortality in patients with gallbladder cancer. Ann Surg Oncol. 2004;11(3):310-5.

7. Miller G, Jarnagin WR. Gallbladder carcinoma. Eur J Surg Oncol. 2008;34(3):306-12.

8. Corvera CU, Blumgart LH, Akhurst T, et al. 18F-fluorodeoxyglucose positron emission tomography influences management decisions in patients with biliary cancer. J Am Coll Surg. 2008;206(1):57-65.

9. Agrawal S, Sonawane RN, Behari A, et al. Laparoscopic staging in gallbladder cancer. Dig Surg. 2005;22(6):440-5.

10. Chan SY, Poon RT, Lo CM, et al. Management of carcinoma of the gallbladder: a single-institution experience in 16 years. J Surg Oncol. 2008;97(2):156-64.

11. Endo I, Shimada H, Tanabe M, et al. Prognostic significance of the number of positive lymph nodes in gallbladder cancer. J Gastrointest Surg. 2006;10(7):999-1007.

12. Liang JW, Dong SX, Zhou ZX, et al. Surgical management for carcinoma of the gallbladder: a single-institution experience in 25 years. Chin Med J. 2008;121(19):1900-5.

13. Shirai Y, Wakai T, Hatakeyama K. Radical lymph node dissection for gallbladder cancer: indications and limitations. Surg Oncol Clin N Am. 2007;16(1):221-32.

14. Kondo S, Nimura Y, Hayakawa N, et al. Extensive surgery for carcinoma of the gallbladder. Br J Surg. 2002;89(2):179-84.

15. Dixon E, Vollmer CM Jr, Sahajpal A, et al. An aggressive surgical approach leads to improved survival in patients with gallbladder cancer: a 12-year study at a North American Center. Ann Surg. 2005;241(3):385-94.

16. Foster JM, Hoshi H, Gibbs JF, et al. Gallbladder cancer: Defining the indications for primary radical resection and radical re-resection. Ann Surg Oncol. 2007;14(2):833-40.

17. Shih SP, Schulick RD, Cameron JL, et al. Gallbladder cancer: the role of laparoscopy and radical resection. Ann Surg. 2007;245(6):893-901.

18. Jayaraman S, Jarnagin WR. Management of gallbladder cancer. Gastroenterol Clin North Am. 2010;39(2):331-42.

19. Wakai T, Shirai Y, Hatakeyama K. Radical second resection provides survival benefit for patients with T2 gallbladder carcinoma first discovered after laparoscopic cholecystectomy. World J Surg. 2002;26(7):867-71.

20. Chijiiwa K, Kai M, Nagano M, et al. Outcome of radical surgery for stage IV gallbladder carcinoma. J Hepatobiliary Pancreat Surg. 2007;14(4):345-50.

21. Kai M, Chijiiwa K, Ohuchida J, et al. A curative resection improves the postoperative survival rate even in patients with advanced gallbladder carcinoma. J Gastrointest Surg. 2007;11(8):1025-32.

22. Kapoor VK. Advanced gallbladder cancer: Indian "middle path". J Hepatobiliary Pancreat Surg. 2007;14(4):366-73.

23. Jensen EH, Abraham A, Jarosek S, et al. Lymph node evaluation is associated with improved survival after surgery for early stage gallbladder cancer. Surgery. 2009;146(4):706-11.

24. Shirai Y, Ohtani T, Tsukada K, et al. Radical surgery is justified for locally advanced gallbladder carcinoma if complete resection is feasible. Am J Gastroenterol. 1997;92(1):181-2.

25. Agarwal AK, Mandal S, Singh S, et al. Gallbladder cancer with duodenal infiltration: is it still resectable? J Gastrointest Surg. 2007;11(12):1722-7.

26. Sasaki R, Takahashi M, Funato O, et al. Hepatopancreatoduodenectomy with wide lymph node dissection for locally advanced carcinoma of the gallbladder—long-term results. Hepatogastroenterology. 2002;49(46):912-5.

27. Araida T, Higuchi R, Hamano M, et al. Should the extrahepatic bile duct be resected or preserved in R0 radical surgery for advanced gallbladder carcinoma? Results of a Japanese Society of Biliary Surgery Survey: a multicenter study. Surg Today. 2009;39(9):770-9.

28. D'Angelica M, Dalal KM, DeMatteo RP, et al. Analysis of the extent of resection for adenocarcinoma of the gallbladder. Ann Surg Oncol. 2009;16(4):806-16.

29. Underwood TJ. Gallbladder Cancer: The rationale for aggressive resection. In: Irving T, Colin DJ. (Eds). Recent Advances in Surgery:33, New Delhi: Jaypee Brothers Medical Publishers (P) Ltd; 2010.

30. Shoup M, Fong Y. Surgical indications and extent of resection in gallbladder cancer. Surg Oncol Clin N Am. 2002;11(4):985-94.

31. Lohe F, Meimarakis G, Schauer C, et al. The time of diagnosis impacts surgical management but not the outcome of patients with gallbladder carcinoma. Eur J Med Res. 2009;14(8):345-51.

32. Kapoor VK, Pradeep R, Haribhakti SP, et al. Intrahepatic segment III cholangiojejunostomy in advanced carcinoma of the gallbladder. Br J Surg. 1996;83(12):1709-11.

33. Czito BG, Hurwitz HI, Clough RW, et al. Adjuvant external-beam radiotherapy with concurrent chemotherapy after resection of primary gallbladder carcinoma: a 23-year experience. Int J Radiat Oncol Biol Phys. 2005;62(4):1030-4.

34. Kayahara M, Nagakawa T. Recent trends of gallbladder cancer in Japan: an analysis of 4,770 patients. Cancer. 2007;110(3):572-80.

35. Lai CH, Lau WY. Gallbladder cancer—a comprehensive review. Surgeon. 2008;6(2):101-10.

36. Cho SY, Kim SH, Park SJ, et al. Adjuvant chemoradiation therapy in gallbladder cancer. J Surg Oncol. 2010;102(1):87-93.

37. de Aretxabala X, Roa I, Berrios M, et al. Chemoradiotherapy in gallbladder cancer. J Surg Oncol. 2006;93(8):699-704.

38. Valle J, Wasan H, Palmer DH, et al. Cisplatin plus gemcitabine versus gemcitabine for biliary tract cancer. N Engl J Med. 2010;362(14):1273-81.
39. Bartlett DL, Fong Y, Fortner JG, et al. Long-term results after resection for gallbladder cancer. Implications for staging and management. Ann Surg. 1996;224(5):639-46.
40. Miura F, Asano T, Amano H, et al. New prognostic factor influencing long-term survival of patients with advanced gallbladder carcinoma. Surgery. 2010;148(2):271-7.
41. Misra S, Chaturvedi A, Misra NC, et al. Carcinoma of the gallbladder. Lancet Oncol. 2003;4(3):167-76.
42. Ong SL, Garcea G, Thomasset SC, et al. Ten-year experience in the management of gallbladder cancer from a single hepatobiliary and pancreatic centre with review of the literature. HPB (Oxford). 2008;10(6):446-58.

CHAPTER SIX

Laparoscopic or Open Liver Resection?

Mirnezami R, Mirnezami AH, Pearce NW

Minimally invasive surgery is increasingly applied to more complex surgical procedures including liver surgery. Nevertheless, studies comparing a laparoscopic technique to open approaches are few and significant concerns exist about morbidity, and long-term oncological outcomes. Here, we summarise the available literature comparing the two techniques and examine the available short-term and long-term outcomes.

EVOLUTION OF LIVER SURGERY

Over the past 30 years liver resection has evolved into an established surgical practice with markedly improved outcomes. Early caution was fuelled by the view that it was high-risk, ineffective and resource-intensive, and combined with concerns regarding high morbidity and mortality, the procedures became limited to only a handful of centres around the world. The remarkable shift in opinion and practice over the past three decades is attributable to several factors. Firstly, there have been significant advances in the understanding of functional and segmental liver anatomy, with the classification systems of Couinaud[1] and Bismuth[2] defining a liver comprised of eight segments. Division of the liver into these 'self-sufficient' units, each with its own vascular inflow, outflow and biliary drainage, has meant that a segment(s) can be resected without causing damage to adjacent units. Secondly, increasingly sophisticated radiological platforms such as contrast-enhanced ultrasound, CT and MRI have provided an unprecedented level of anatomical detail, allowing accurate assessment of tumour location and extent, and proximity to major vascular/biliary structures. Thirdly, ongoing research efforts have resulted in an enhanced understanding of the natural history of primary and metastatic liver tumours, leading to a growing conviction that radical treatment can result in improved cancer related outcomes. In addition, refinements in anaesthesia and critical care have greatly assisted more complex surgery on the liver with fewer complications. Finally, liver

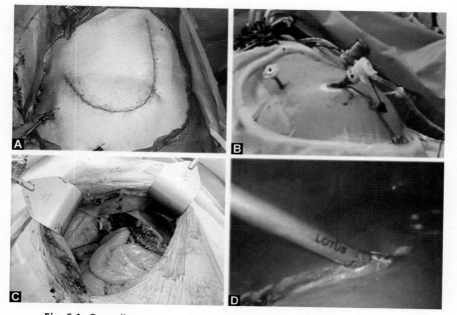

Fig. 6.1: Open (images A and C) and laparoscopic (images B and D) liver surgery are increasingly conducted worldwide

resection for malignant tumours is now further facilitated by the increasing use of chemotherapeutic agents to 'downstage' initially unresectable disease and allow for subsequent, potentially curative surgery to be undertaken. Thus, in patients in whom disease is confined to the liver, it is estimated that currently used chemotherapeutic regimes can convert up to 30 to 40 per cent of cases to resectable disease.[3] For all these reasons, liver resection is increasingly performed in specialist centres around the world (Fig. 6.1).

Key Point

- Improved understanding of segmental liver anatomy together with radiological, technical and critical care improvements have allowed liver resection to become an established part of surgical practice over the past 30 years.

LAPAROSCOPIC LIVER RESECTION: THE NEXT PARADIGM

Beginning in the late 1980s with cholecystectomy, operative surgery of the gastrointestinal tract has been revolutionised by minimally invasive techniques. The laparoscopic approach is now regarded as the 'gold standard' for a variety of increasingly complex procedures including cholecystectomy,[4] appendicectomy,[5] anti-reflux surgery[6] and more recently colorectal resection.[7] Advantages of laparoscopy over conventional open surgery include reduced postoperative pain, enhanced cosmetic outcome and shorter length of hospital stay, and have been demonstrated across a variety of surgical subspecialties.

By comparison, liver surgeons have been somewhat slow to embrace the laparoscopic movement. Gagner and colleagues reported the first case of laparoscopic liver resection (LLR) for benign disease in 1992,[8] and the first report of LLR for malignancy was published by Wayand and Woisetschlager soon afterward in 1994.[9] These early reports confirmed the feasibility of LLR and since then approximately 3,000 cases of LLR have been performed worldwide for varying indications including benign tumours, colorectal liver metastases and hepatocellular carcinoma (HCC).[10] Although LLR is steadily growing, it has yet to gain widespread acceptance.[10] Several explanations are likely to account for this. Firstly, from a technical perspective, liver mobilisation and parenchymal transection can be difficult laparoscopically, and haemorrhage arguably the most feared hazard in liver resection can also present a significant challenge laparoscopically.[11,12] In addition, there is the theoretical risk of gas embolism during division of the hepatic veins under pneumoperitoneum.[13] The arduous learning curve and concerns regarding the ease with which the necessary skills can be disseminated amongst liver surgeons constitute further reservations. Technical considerations aside, there also remains uncertainty regarding the adequacy of oncological resection with LLR when compared to conventional open liver resection (OLR) for malignancy.

Key Point

- Perceived difficulties with liver mobilisation, parenchymal transection, haemorrhage control and the potential for gas embolism have meant that laparoscopic liver resection has been slow to gain acceptance compared with other surgical subspecialties.

INDICATIONS AND CASE SELECTION

The indications for LLR do not differ significantly from those for OLR and continue to evolve. Symptomatic benign tumours or those that are of indeterminate nature should be considered for resection and it is at this point a laparoscopic approach should be considered if appropriate. In terms of malignant disease, as with OLR, the main indications for LLR are colorectal cancer metastases (CRCM) and hepatocellular carcinoma (HCC). In general, laparoscopic approach is not considered suitable for gallbladder cancers and hilar cholangiocarcinomas for fear of peritoneal tumour dissemination, and the need for hilar dissection.[14,15] However, each case needs to be judged individually and the authors are aware of successful management of early and predicted node-negative gallbladder cancers, and some peri-hilar cholangiocarcinomas by a minimally invasive technique at ours and other units, illustrating the evolving nature of the indications.

However, the threshold for intervention may prove different; thus, in patients with symptomatic benign disease, diagnostic doubt, or in those undergoing palliative cytoreduction, the lower physical insult of laparoscopic surgery may provide an impetus for earlier consideration of surgical options as evidenced by the high proportion of patients undergoing resection for benign disease in most published case series.

Irrespective of indication for surgery, the two most frequently reported selection criteria for LLR are tumour location and tumour size. With respect to location, it is generally agreed that tumours located in the left and/or anterolateral Couinaud segments (segments 2–6), and planned for subsegmental/segmental resections or left lateral sectionectomy are best suited to the laparoscopic approach.[16] Laparoscopic resection for lesions involving segments 1, 7 and 8 are technically more challenging and the feasibility of these resections by laparoscopic means has yet to be clearly demonstrated. Other selection criteria that have been proposed include tumour size not exceeding 5 cm in maximal diameter,[17] first time liver resection,[18] resection in patients with noncirrhotic livers or child's A or B stage cirrhosis,[19] ASA grade less than or equal to three,[20] and tumours not associated with any major vascular or biliary involvement.[20] Nevertheless these criteria are likely to change with technological advances, better instrumentation and increasing experience with minimally invasive techniques, and the senior author has experience of successful resections despite the described contraindications.

Key Point

- The laparoscopic approach is currently best suited to tumours located in the left/anterolateral Couinaud segments (2–6).

EVALUATION OF LAPAROSCOPIC LIVER RESECTION: IS THE EVIDENCE THERE?

To date, there has been no randomised controlled trial (RCT) to compare outcomes between LLR and OLR. Indeed, while a well conducted RCT comparing the two approaches would be desirable; it may prove unethical to randomise patients in some centres with a large experience of LLR. Therefore, recently available evidence consists of case series or comparative studies, where results have been compared with those achieved with OLR. These studies have demonstrated the feasibility of LLR; however, caution must be exerted when interpreting the results from such reports, as most LLR have been performed at large tertiary centres with skilled surgeons in advanced laparoscopic surgery and where **75** practices, and patient selection strategies vary considerably. Furthermore, while most studies have evaluated short-term outcomes with LLR and OLR, relatively few studies have assessed long-term oncological outcomes, and this is an area that is likely to require further study before firm conclusions can be drawn.

Key Point

- There is no high quality evidence comparing LLR and OLR at present.

SHORT-TERM OUTCOMES

Since Rau, et al. performed the first study comparing short-term outcomes with LLR and OLR in 1998,[21] there have been over 30 further publications in the English literature aiming to clarify the situation. Table 6.1 summarises the findings of 18 recent studies comparing short-term outcomes for LLR versus OLR (from 2005 onwards). The combined population from these studies is 1,278 (range 20–179). Laparoscopic resection was performed in 571 patients (45%) and open resection in 707 (55%). The cumulative conversion-to-open rate for all laparoscopic procedures presented here was 8 per cent (45 out of 571). Thirty day mortality occurred in 0.5 per cent of patients undergoing LLR (3 out of 571) compared with 1 per cent of patients undergoing OLR (8 out of 707). The reported incidence of gas embolism with LLR was 0.2 per cent (1 out of 571).

With respect to perioperative outcomes, the results suggest that LLR takes longer to perform compared with conventional open surgery. However, in keeping with trends observed in other subspecialties, it is likely that as experience with LLR increases the procedure duration will shorten. Indeed, it is even conceivable that in future LLR may take less time than OLR, since the latter involves larger and more time consuming incisions.

The other consistent findings from the studies summarised in Table 6.1 are that laparoscopic liver resection results in otherwise favourable short-term outcomes including reduced operative blood loss and shorter length of hospital stay. Several authors have found a quicker return to oral intake and a reduced rate of postoperative complications. A meta-analysis of 8 studies performed by Simillis, et al. in 2007 compared short-term outcomes between LLR and OLR, and found LLR to be associated with reduced blood loss, duration of portal triad clamping and duration of hospital stay, and a quicker time to first oral intake.[22]

The issue of haemorrhage warrants particular attention, since intra-operative bleeding during liver parenchymal transection is of great concern, and the reported incidence is 7 per cent in the literature.[23] Early studies suggested that LLR results in reduced blood loss after minor liver resections[24] and left lateral sectionectomies.[25] However, it has been unclear, if this finding would also apply to more complex resections. Dagher, et al. recently reported on outcomes in closely matched patients undergoing right hepatectomy. In their study of 72 patients, they found blood loss to be reduced with LLR compared with OLR (519 ml+/-93 and 735 ml+/-74 respectively; p=0.038).[20] Although few surgeons would counsel against conversion in the face of major haemorrhage the increasingly sophisticated array of available laparoscopic equipment for control of bleeding may support more complex surgery, a view reiterated in a recent multinational consensus conference examining the role of LLR.[26]

At the present time, data relating to cost outcomes with LLR and OLR is limited. Polignano, et al. reported increased costs of disposable instrument with LLR compared with OLR. However, these expenses were offset by reduced high care and ward stay costs; and total costs were significantly lower with LLR.[27] Similarly, Tsinberg and colleagues also reported significantly reduced hospital and overall costs with LLR compared with OLR.[28] These are encouraging findings and particularly of value in view of current economic constraints.

> ## Key Point
>
> - LLR is associated with increased procedure times but otherwise favourable short-term outcomes including reduced blood loss, shorter hospital stay and quicker return to oral intake.

LAPAROSCOPIC LIVER RESECTION FOR MALIGNANT DISEASE

Several studies have compared the outcomes of LLR and OLR for malignant disease and their findings are discussed below according to the primary tumour concerned. Key findings have been summarised in Tables 6.2 and 6.3.

Colorectal Liver Metastases

Data specifically evaluating LLR for CRLM is somewhat limited and until recently, has been largely reliant on noncomparative studies. Nguyen, et al. reported oncological outcomes from a large multiinstitutional cohort of patients undergoing LLR for CRLM and found that resection margin status and overall 5-year survival were comparable with data from contemporary open series.[10] Mala, et al. performed the first study specifically comparing open and laparoscopic liver resection for CRLM in 2002.[43] The authors reported equivalent resection margin status but no survival data were provided. Studies by Castaing, et al.[41] and Abu Hilal, et al.[44] have also demonstrated equivalent resection margin and survival outcomes for patients undergoing LLR compared with OLR. Table 6.2 provides summary data from these comparative studies.

TABLE 6.1

Summary of most recent series comparing short-term outcomes for LLR and OLR (2005 onwards)

Reference	Year	No. of patients LLR/OLR	% Conversion	30-day mortality	% Major resections LLR/OLR[†]	Perioperative (LLR vs. OLR) outcomes
Kaneko, et al.[29]	2005	30/28	3	–	0/0	→ OT; ↓ BL; ↓ LOS*; ↓ TRD*; ↓↔ POC
Aldrighetti, et al.[30]	2008	20/20	–	–	0/0	↑ OT (NS); ↓ BL*; ↓ LOS*; ↓ POC
Polignano, et al.[27]	2008	25/25	8	–	0/0	↓ OT (NS); ↓ BL*; ↓ LOS*; ↓ POC*
Troisi, et al.[31]	2008	20/20	1		5/10	↓ OT (NS); ↓ LOS*; ↓ TRD*
Lee, et al.[32]	2007	25/25	8		0/0	↑ OT (NS); ↓ BL*; ↓ LOS*; ↓ TRD*; ↔POC
Abu Hilal, et al.[33]	2008	24/20	–		0/0	↑ OT (NS); ↓ BL*; ↓ LOS*; ↓ POC (NS)
Topal, et al.[34]	2008	76/76	9		28/NA	↓OT*; ↓ BL*; ↓ LOS*
Cai, et al.[35]	2009	19/19	11		100/100	↑ OT (NS); ↓ BL*; ↓ LOS (NS); ↔ POC
Sarpel, et al.[36]	2009	20/56	–		NA	↓ OT (NS); ↓ LOS; ↓ POC (NS)
Tranchart, et al.[19]	2010	42/42	5	LLR (1) OLR (1)	12/12	↑ OT (NS); ↓ BL*; ↓ LOS*; ↓ POC (NS)
Tsinberg, et al.[28]	2009	31/43	–	–	0/0	↑ OT (NS); ↓ BL*; ↓ LOS*; ↓ TRD*
Rowe, et al.[37]	2009	18/12	6	–	6/0	↓ OT (NS);↓ BL*; ↓ LOS*; ↓ POC*
Ito, et al.[38]	2009	65/65	20	–	0/0	↑ OT*; ↓BL*; ↓LOS*; ↓ TRD*; ↓ POC*
Endo, et al.[39]	2009	10/11	–	–	0/0	↑ OT (NS); ↑ BL (NS); ↓ LOS*; ↓ TRD*; ↓ POC*
Dagher, et al.[20]	2009	22/50	9	LLR (0) OLR (1)	100/100	↑ OT (NS); ↓ BL*; ↓ LOS*; ↓ POC*
Carswell, et al.[40]	2009	10/10	10	–	0/0	↑ OT (NS); ↓ LOS*
Castaing, et al.[41]	2009	60/60	10	LLR (1) OLR (1)	52/45	↓ BL*; ↓ LOS (NS); ↓ POC (NS)
Belli, et al.[42]	2009	54/125	7	LLR (1) OLR (5)	6/31	↓ OT*; ↓ BL*; ↓ LOS (NS); ↓ POC*

* statistically significant (p<0.05); **BL** blood loss; **NS** not statistically significant; **LOS** length of stay; **NA** not available; **POC** postoperative complication; **DFS** disease-free survival; **TRD** time to resumption of diet; **OT** operating time; **LLR** laparoscopic liver resection; OLR open liver resection; procedure classed as major resection where ≥ 3 segments resected

† **LLR** laparoscopic liver resection; OLR open liver resection; procedure classed as major resection where ≥ 3 segments resected

TABLE 6.2

Studies comparing oncological outcome with LLR versus OLR for colorectal cancer metastases

Reference	Year	No. of patients LLR/OLR	Resection margin	% positive margins	Disease recurrence	Overall survival	Disease-free survival
Mala, et al.[43]	2002	21/14	LLR ≥1cm in 71% OLR ≥1cm in 63%	LLR 5% OLR 14%	NA[†] NA	NA NA	NA NA
Castaing, et al.[41]	2009	60/60	LLR 5.3 mm OLR 5.2 mm	LLR 13% OLR 28%[*]	LLR 57% OLR 70%	LLR at 5-yr 64% OLR at 5-yr 56%	LLR at 5-yr 30% OLR at 5-yr 20%
Abu Hilal, et al.[44]	2010	50/85	LLR 17.3 mm OLR NA	LLR 4% OLR 6%	LLR 16% OLR 17.6%	LLR at 30-mth 90% OLR at 30-mth 58%	NA NA

* statistically significant (p<0.05)

† NA data not available

TABLE 6.3

Studies comparing oncological outcome with LLR versus OLR for hepatocellular carcinoma

Reference	Year	No. of patients LLR/OLR	Resection margin	% positive margins	Disease recurrence	Overall survival	Disease-free survival
Shimada, et al.[18]	2001	17/38	LLR 8 mm OLR 7 mm	LLR 41% OLR 50%	NA[†] NA	LLR at 5-yr 47% OLR at 5-yr 34%	LLR at 5-yr 41% OLR at 5-yr 54%
Lesurtel, et al.[25]	2003	13/14	LLR 9 mm OLR 8.8 mm		LLR 38% OLR 50%	LLR at 3-yr 89% OLR at 3-yr 55% *	LLR at 3-yr 50% OLR at 3-yr 48%
Kaneko, et al.[29]	2005	30/28	NA	NA	NA	LLR at 5-yr 61% OLR at 5-yr 62%	LLR at 5-yr 31% OLR at 5-yr 29%
Sarpel, et al.[36]	2009	20/56	NA	LLR 10% OLR 27%	LLR 52% OLR 46%	LLR at 5-yr 91% OLR at 5-yr 78%	NA
Tranchart, et al.[19]	2010	42/42	LLR 10.4 mm OLR 10.6 mm	NA	LLR 24% OLR 29%	LLR at 5-yr 60% OLR at 5-yr 47%	LLR at 5-yr 46% OLR at 5-yr 37%
Endo, et al.[39]	2009	10/11	LLR 17 mm OLR 17 mm	NA	NA	LLR at 5-yr 57% OLR at 5-yr 48%	LLR at 5-yr 24% OLR at 5-yr 19%
Belli, et al.[42]	2009	54/125	NA	LLR 0% OLR 6%	LLR 45% OLR 53%	LLR at 36-mth 67% OLR at 36-mth 60%	LLR at 36-mth 52% OLR at 36-mth 59%
Aldrighetti, et al.[50]	2010	16/16	NA	NA	NA	LLR at 32-mth 40% OLR at 32-mth 48%	LLR at 32-mth 23% OLR at 32-mth 31%

* statistically significant (p<0.05)

† NA data not available

In 2010, Welsh and colleagues published a large series on outcomes in patients undergoing OLR for CRLM.[45] They compared long-term outcomes in 266 OLR cases which were deemed suitable for LLR with 886 OLR cases not deemed suitable for LLR. The authors found higher rates of resection margin involvement and lower disease-free survival rates in cases not suitable for LLR. They explained this finding by suggesting that LLR selects for patients who have more favourable disease, who require relatively simpler resections with less risk of margin involvement and better overall survival. This finding again highlights the fact that results comparing cancer related outcomes with LLR and OLR should be interpreted with care.

Hepatocellular Carcinoma

With respect to HCC, eight studies have reported comparative oncological outcome data for LLR and OLR and this data is summarised in Table 6.3. These studies demonstrate equivalent results in terms of margin status, disease recurrence and overall disease-free survival with LLR in comparison to OLR. Special mention is warranted in the case of cirrhotic patients undergoing OLR for HCC, where postoperative ascites and hepatic decompensation can pose significant difficulties. As the abdominal wall is relatively spared from injury in LLR, this may reduce any loss of collateral venous circulation when compared to open surgical incisions and potentially limit postoperative rises in portal pressure. In support of this, some studies have noted a significant increase in postoperative cirrhotic decompensation with OLR compared to LLR.[19] Further studies are necessary to evaluate this finding in more detail. Laparoscopic liver resection may also be advantageous in cases of HCC complicating established chronic liver disease. Liver transplantation remains the main strategy in these patients; however this is frequently preceded by liver resection or radiofrequency ablation for disease control, because of the given shortage of donor livers. Recent reports have suggested that liver transplantation after previous laparotomy is technically more difficult and associated with significant blood loss.[46] Laurent and colleagues evaluated procedure duration and blood loss with liver transplantation after previous LLR or OLR.[47] Patients who had LLR as the first procedure had shorter operating times and reduced blood loss, suggesting that LLR may facilitate the transplant procedure.

One area of potential concern that has been raised about minimally invasive surgery for cancer has been the possibility of peritoneal seeding and port site recurrence. While this has been addressed by several large scale RCTs in other surgical sub-specialties,[48] it has not been examined in liver surgery specifically. From the studies depicted in Tables 6.2 and 6.3, no reported cases of port-site recurrence following LLR for malignant disease have been described, suggesting that this is likely to be a rare occurrence.

Interestingly, proponents of a minimally invasive approach have suggested that laparoscopic surgery may actually be oncologically superior to conventional open surgery. Thus, experimental studies have shown that open surgery results in increased systemic levels of circulatory cytokines and growth factors implicated in tumour growth, survival and proliferation.[49] In addition, enhanced recovery and reduced postoperative complications following laparoscopic surgery may facilitate early institution of adjuvant therapy, which may further improve cancer outcomes.

Key Point

- Although limited, current reports suggest equivalent short-term cancer related outcomes when comparing LLR and OLR.

CONCLUSION

The available literature constitutes observational studies with significant limitations and there is a lack of high quality evidence to draw conclusions from them. The data presented must be interpreted with caution and primarily originates from large, tertiary centres with potentially significant differences in case mix, protocol, and surgical expertise. Low conversion and perioperative mortality rates in the described LLR groups also suggests that cases were accomplished by experienced surgeons with advanced laparoscopic skills who have already ascended their learning curves, thereby limiting generalisability.

Nevertheless, the data highlights the feasibility and safety of LLR. In experienced hands and in appropriately selected cases, LLR results in favourable short-term outcomes including reduced operative blood loss, shorter duration of hospital stay and earlier resumption of oral intake. For malignant disease, although few comparative studies have been conducted, analysis of cancer related outcomes for CRLM and HCC suggest seemingly equivalent oncological results. These findings are also in line with evidence that has accumulated from large scale multicentre randomised studies on the use of laparoscopic colorectal surgery for malignant pathology.[7,48,51,52] Further studies will help to clarify this and allow the role of LLR in future practice to be defined more precisely.

Key Points for Clinical Practice

- Improved understanding of segmental liver anatomy together with radiological, technical and critical care improvements have allowed liver resection to become an established part of surgical practice over the past 30 years.
- Perceived difficulties with liver mobilisation, parenchymal transection, haemorrhage control and the potential for gas embolism have meant that laparoscopic liver resection has been slow to gain acceptance compared with other surgical subspecialties.
- The laparoscopic approach is currently best suited to tumours located in the left/anterolateral Couinaud segments (2–6).
- There is no high quality evidence comparing LLR and OLR at present.
- LLR is associated with increased procedure times but otherwise favourable short-term outcomes including reduced blood loss, shorter hospital stay and quicker return to oral intake.
- Although limited, current reports suggest equivalent short-term cancer related outcomes when comparing LLR and OLR.

REFERENCES

1. Lafortune M, Madore F, Patriquin H, et al. Segmental anatomy of the liver: a sonographic approach to the Couinaud nomenclature. Radiology 1991;181(2):443-8.
2. Bismuth H. Surgical anatomy and anatomical surgery of the liver. World J Surg 1982;6(1):3-9.
3. Homayounfar K, Liersch T, Niessner M, et al. Multimodal treatment options for bilobar colorectal liver metastases. Langenbecks Arch Surg 2010;395(6):633-41.
4. Keus F, de Jong JA, Gooszen HG, et al. Laparoscopic versus open cholecystectomy for patients with symptomatic cholecystolithiasis. Cochrane Database Syst Rev 2006;18(4):CD006231.
5. Bennett J, Boddy A, Rhodes M. Choice of approach for appendicectomy: a meta-analysis of open versus laparoscopic appendicectomy. Surg Laparosc Endosc Percutan Tech 2007;17(4):245-55.
6. Jamieson GG, Watson DI, Britten-Jones R, et al. Laparoscopic Nissen fundoplication. Ann Surg 1994;220:137-45.
7. Jayne DG, Guillou PJ, Thorpe H, et al. Randomized trial of laparoscopic-assisted resection of colorectal carcinoma: 3-year results of the UK MRC CLASICC Trial Group. J Clin Oncol 2007;25(21):3061-8.
8. Gagner M, Rheault M, Dubuc J. Laparoscopic partial hepatectomy for liver tumor. Surg Endosc 1992;6:97-8.
9. Wayand W, Woisetschlager R. Laparoscopic resection of liver metastasis. Chirurg 1993;64:195-7.

10. Nguyen KT, Laurent A, Dagher I, et al. Minimally invasive liver resection for metastatic colorectal cancer: a multi-institutional, international report of safety, feasibility, and early outcomes. Ann Surg 2009;250(5):842-8.

11. Dagher I, O'Rourke N, Geller DA, et al. Laparoscopic major hepatectomy: an evolution in standard of care. Ann Surg 2009;250(5):856-60.

12. Bryant R, Laurent A, Tayar C, et al. Laparoscopic liver resection— understanding its role in current practice: The Henri Mondor Hospital experience. Ann Surg 2009;250(1):103-11.

13. Schmandra TC, Mierdl S, Bauer H, et al. Transoesophageal echocardiography shows high risk of gas embolism during laparoscopic hepatic resection under carbon dioxide pneumoperitoneum. Br J Surg 2002;89(7):870-6.

14. Fong Y, Brennan MF, Turnbull A, et al. Gallbladder cancer discovered during laparoscopic surgery. Potential for iatrogenic tumor dissemination. Arch Surg 1993;128(9):1054-6.

15. Johnstone PA, Rohde DC, Swartz SE, et al. Port site recurrences after laparoscopic and thoracoscopic procedures in malignancy. J Clin Oncol 1996;14(6):1950-6.

16. Cherqui D. Laparoscopic liver resection. Br J Surg 2003;90(6):644-6.

17. Dagher I, Proske JM, Carloni A, et al. Laparoscopic liver resection: results for 70 patients. Surg Endosc 2007;21(4):619-24.

18. Shimada M, Hashizume M, Maehara S, et al. Laparoscopic hepatectomy for hepatocellular carcinoma. Surg Endosc 2001;15:541-4.

19. Tranchart H, Di Giuro G, Lainas P, et al. Laparoscopic resection for hepatocellular carcinoma: a matched-pair comparative study. Surg Endosc 2010; 24(5):1170-6.

20. Dagher I, Di Giuro G, Dubrez J, et al. Laparoscopic versus open right hepatectomy: a comparative study. Am J Surg 2009;198(2):173-7.

21. Rau HG, Buttler E, Meyer G, et al. Laparoscopic liver resection compared with conventional partial hepatectomy—a prospective analysis. Hepatogastroenterology 1998;45(24):2333-8.

22. Simillis C, Constantinides VA, Tekkis PP, et al. Laparoscopic versus open hepatic resections for benign and malignant neoplasms—a meta-analysis. Surgery 2007;141(2):203-11.

23. Chen HY, Juan CC, Ker CG. Laparoscopic liver surgery for patients with hepatocellular carcinoma. Ann Surg Oncol 2008;15(3):800-6.

24. Morino M, Morra I, Rosso E, et al. Laparoscopic versus open hepatic resection: a comparative study. Surg Endosc 2003;17:1914-8.

25. Lesurtel M, Cherqui D, Laurent A, et al. Laparoscopic versus open left lateral hepatic lobectomy: a case-control study. J Am Coll Surg 2003;196(2):236-42.

26. Buell JF, Cherqui D, Geller DA, et al. The international position on laparoscopic liver surgery: The Louisville Statement, 2008. Ann Surg 2009;250(5):825-30.

27. Polignano FM, Quyn AJ, de Figueiredo RS, et al. Laparoscopic versus open liver segmentectomy: prospective, case-matched, intention-to-treat analysis of clinical outcomes and cost effectiveness. Surg Endosc 2008;22(12):2564-70.

28. Tsinberg M, Tellioglu G, Simpfendorfer CH, et al. Comparison of laparoscopic versus open liver tumor resection: a case-controlled study. Surg Endosc 2009;23(4):847-53.

29. Kaneko H, Takagi S, Otsuka Y, et al. Laparoscopic liver resection of hepatocellular carcinoma. Am J Surg 2005;189(2):190-4.

30. Aldrighetti L, Pulitanò C, Catena M, et al. A prospective evaluation of laparoscopic versus open left lateral hepatic sectionectomy. J Gastrointest Surg 2008;12(3):457-62.

31. Troisi R, Montalti R, Smeets P, et al. The value of laparoscopic liver surgery for solid benign hepatic tumors. Surg Endosc. 2008;22(1):38-44.

32. Lee KF, Cheung YS, Chong CN, et al. Laparoscopic versus open hepatectomy for liver tumours: a case-control study. Hong Kong Med J 2007;13(6):442-8.

33. Abu Hilal M, McPhail MJ, Zeidan B, et al. Laparoscopic versus open left lateral hepatic sectionectomy: A comparative study. Eur J Surg Oncol 2008; 34(12):1285-8.

34. Topal B, Fieuws S, Aerts R, et al. Laparoscopic versus open liver resection of hepatic neoplasms: comparative analysis of short-term results. Surg Endosc 2008;22(10):2208-13.

35. Cai XJ, Wang YF, Liang YL, et al. Laparoscopic left hemihepatectomy: A safety and feasibility study of 19 cases. Surg Endosc 2009;23(11):2556-62.

36. Sarpel U, Hefti MM, Wisnievsky JP, et al. Outcome for patients treated with laparoscopic versus open resection of hepatocellular carcinoma: case-matched analysis. Ann Surg Oncol 2009;16(6):1572-7.

37. Rowe AJ, Meneghetti AT, Schumacher PA, et al. Perioperative analysis of laparoscopic versus open liver resection. Surg Endosc 2009;23(6):1198-203.

38. Ito K, Ito H, Are C, et al. Laparoscopic versus open liver resection: a matched-pair case control study. J Gastrointest Surg 2009;13(12):2276-83.

39. Endo Y, Ohta M, Sasaki A, et al. A comparative study of the long-term outcomes after laparoscopy-assisted and open left lateral hepatectomy for hepatocellular carcinoma. Surg Laparosc Endosc Percutan Tech 2009;19(5):171-4.

40. Carswell KA, Sagias FG, Murgatroyd B, et al. Laparoscopic versus open left lateral segmentectomy. BMC Surg 2009;9:14.

41. Castaing D, Vibert E, Ricca L, et al. Oncologic results of laparoscopic versus open hepatectomy for colorectal liver metastases in two specialised centres. Ann Surg 2009;250(5):849-55.

42. Belli G, Limongelli P, Fantini C, et al. Laparoscopic and open treatment of hepatocellular carcinoma in patients with cirrhosis. Br J Surg 2009;96(9): 1041-8.

43. Mala T, Edwin B, Gladhaug I, et al. A comparative study of the short-term outcome following open and laparoscopic liver resection of colorectal metastases. Surg Endosc 2002;16(7):1059-63.

44. Abu Hilal M, Underwood T, Zuccaro M, et al. Short- and medium-term results of totally laparoscopic resection for colorectal liver metastases. Br J Surg 2010;97(6):927-33.

45. Welsh FK, Tekkis PP, John TG, et al. Open liver resection for colorectal metastases: better short- and long-term outcomes in patients potentially suitable for laparoscopic liver resection. HPB (Oxford) 2010;12(3):188-94.

46. Adam R, Azoulay D. Is primary resection and salvage transplantation for hepatocellular carcinoma a reasonable strategy? Ann Surg 2005;241(4): 671-2.

47. Laurent A, Tayar C, Andreoletti M, et al. Laparoscopic liver resection facilitates salvage liver transplantation for hepatocellular carcinoma. J Hepatobiliary Pancreat Surg. 2009;16(3):310-4.

48. Lacy AM, Garcia-Valdecasas JC, Delgado S, et al. Laparoscopy-assisted colectomy versus open colectomy for treatment of non-metastatic colon cancer: a randomised trial. Lancet. 2002;359(9325):2224-9.

49. Novitsky YW, Litwin DE, Callery MP. The net immunologic advantage of laparoscopic surgery. Surg Endosc 2004;18:1411-19.

50. Aldrighetti L, Guzzetti E, Pulitanò C, et al. Case-matched analysis of totally laparoscopic versus open liver resection for HCC: Short and middle term results. J Surg Oncol 2010;102(1):82-6.

51. Clinical Outcomes of Surgical Therapy Study Group. A comparison of laparoscopically-assisted and open colectomy for colon cancer. N Engl J Med 2004;350(20):2050-9.

52. Colon Cancer Laparoscopic or Open Resection Study Group, Buunen M, Veldkamp R, et al. Survival after laparoscopic surgery versus open surgery for colon cancer: Long-term outcome of a randomised clinical trial. Lancet Oncol 2009;10(1):44-52.

CHAPTER SEVEN

Volume and Outcome in Upper Gastrointestinal Malignancy

Richard JE Skipworth, Simon Paterson-Brown

INTRODUCTION

Over the last few years, there has been an increasing recognition that both hospital and surgeon volume have an important role to play in the outcome of patients undergoing complex surgical procedures. Higher hospital volume is associated with reduced postoperative mortality following colectomy,[1] pelvic exenteration,[2] pneumonectomy,[2] paediatric cardiac surgery,[3] carotid endarterectomy[4] and abdominal aortic aneurysm repair,[5] when compared with lower volume hospitals. In the field of upper gastrointestinal (GI) surgery, the volume-outcome relationship (VOR) has been investigated in procedures for both malignant and benign disease. From a benign perspective, high volume (HV) centres have reported both lower mortality and higher rates of successful endoscopic intervention in patients with non-variceal upper GI haemorrhage;[6] and in patients undergoing bariatric surgery, higher hospital volume was associated with a shorter length of stay, decreased rates of morbidity and mortality, and decreased costs.[7] In benign paediatric upper GI surgery, a study of 11,003 patients with hypertrophic pyloric stenosis demonstrated a higher rate of postoperative complications for both low volume (LV) hospitals and surgeons,[8] compared with HV counterparts.

There are now a large number of reported studies that have examined the role of volume in malignant upper GI surgery, with the majority confirming a positive VOR. Such studies have represented one of the drivers towards the centralisation of care for upper GI cancer that is now common practice in many parts of the world. In California between 1990 and 1994, 88 per cent of oesophagectomies were performed in hospitals that carried out only one or two resections per year.[9] Subsequent National US data showed that postoperative mortality rates for oesophagectomy were 20.3 per cent if a centre performed less than two resections per year, compared with 8.4 per cent if more than 19 resections were performed per year. Similar data were demonstrated for gastrectomy (mortality rate 11.4% if <5 resections/year, but 8.6% if >21) and pancreatic resections (mortality rate 16.3% if <1 resections/year, but 3.8% if >16).[10]

Though it is true to say that some LV hospitals (and surgeons) have demonstrated comparable results to HV counterparts, this has often been from small enthusiastic centres and may be related, in part, to very tight case selection. Furthermore, these results have not been reproduced consistently in independent multi-centre studies or national audit figures. Therefore, it would probably be fair to say that the era of the 'part-time resectionist' is now in the past. The problem at present is defining the appropriate resection numbers for HV centres and surgeons. There are obvious significant political and financial implications in developing any such definitions and the associated reorganisation of surgical services.

This chapter will examine in more detail the relationship between volume and outcome in malignant upper GI resectional surgery (including oesophageal, gastric, pancreatic and liver resections) with regard to both individual hospital and surgeon variables.

HOSPITAL VOLUME AND UPPER GI CANCER SURGERY

In a systematic review of VOR studies by Chowdhury, et al. which incorporated 42 different surgical procedures and spanned 13 surgical specialities (n=163 studies included), 74 per cent of hospital volume studies were found to demonstrate a positive VOR.[11] A further cancer-specific systematic review (n=68 studies reviewed; n=41 included) concluded that all studies demonstrated evidence of an inverse relationship between provider volume and postoperative mortality.[12] Although not specific to upper GI cancer, both of these analyses confirm hospital volume as a key determinant of patient outcome in many disease processes.

Some reports have extended their analysis of HV versus LV centres to include an assessment of hospital 'quality' by considering teaching status, university affiliation, recognition by national bodies and even ownership. In Ontario, Canada, the 5-year relative survival of patients following oesophagectomy was 49.2 per cent in University hospitals compared with 32.6 per cent and 27.3 per cent for non-University and non-teaching hospitals respectively.[13] Those hospitals recognised as regional centres of excellence by the National Cancer Institute (NCI) had lower adjusted postoperative mortality rates for oesophagectomy and gastrectomy than those treated at comparable HV hospitals but similar long-term survival.[14] However, of the different definitions of hospital volume used, it is not known currently which is the most influential on patient outcome. In one unadjusted analysis, the benefit of oesophageal, pancreatic and hepatic resections seen in teaching hospitals was removed once adjustment for hospital volume was performed,[15] implying that procedural volume is more important than academic status.

Key Points

- Many studies have suggested that hospital volume and surgeon volume are both key determinants of outcome following oesophageal, gastric, pancreatic and liver resections.
- It is unclear as to whether hospital volume or surgeon volume is the more important determinant of outcome.

SPECIFIC AREAS WHERE HOSPITAL VOLUME INFLUENCES OUTCOME

Staging in Upper GI Malignancy

In a Dutch study of patients with oesophageal cancer (n=573), preoperative staging investigations were repeated or re-evaluated in one central HV referral centre. Whereas true-positive malignant lymph nodes and metastases were detected in 7 per cent and 8 per cent of patients respectively in LV regional hospitals; the HV centre found true-positive malignant lymph nodes and metastases in 16 per cent and 20 per cent respectively.[16] Thus, in 13 per cent of patients at least one metastatic deposit had been missed, so that even allowing for resectability of M1a lymph nodes, inappropriate resections had been planned in 6 per cent of patients. The authors concluded that the reasons for the more accurate staging in the HV centre could, in part, be the result of superior CT equipment but the greater experience of the radiologist was also likely to be important.

Quality of Surgery

There have been several reports that support the view that HV centres carry out more radical/potentially curative surgery. One study comparing patients undergoing gastrectomy and pancreatectomy in National Comprehensive Cancer Network (NCNN), NCI-recognised hospitals and HV centres with community hospitals, and LV centres demonstrated that those in the former groups had a higher number of lymph nodes evaluated.[17] In another study of gastric adenocarcinoma, pathological assessment of more than 15 nodes was only seen in 31 per cent of community hospital resected specimens compared with 38 per cent in teaching hospitals (p<0.01).[18] Furthermore, modern surgical techniques such as laparoscopic resection and endoscopic ultrasonography were more common in the teaching centres. In yet another study, involved resection margins were more likely to be seen following pancreatectomy in LV hospitals compared with HV counterparts.[19]

Postoperative Complications

The rates of postoperative renal failure, pulmonary failure, aspiration, re-intubation, septicaemia, and overall surgical complications were all

89

significantly higher at LV hospitals compared with HV following oesophageal resection.[20] Other studies have also demonstrated fewer cardiac and haemorrhagic complications in HV centres.[21]

Postoperative Mortality

In-hospital mortality is the most commonly examined outcome in VOR studies and has been assessed on a nationwide scale in various countries. Hollenbeck, et al. used data from the USA Nationwide Inpatient Sample between 1993 and 2003 to show that the mortality rates for patients undergoing upper GI resection were significantly higher in LV centres (bottom decile) compared with HV centres (top decile) for oesophagectomy (14.9% vs. 4.8%; adjusted odds ratio [OR] of mortality 2.2; 95% confidence interval [CI] 1.3–3.5), pancreatectomy (11.8% vs. 1.7%; adjusted OR 4.9; 95% CI 2.4–10.1) and liver resection (13.5% vs. 5.7%; adjusted OR 2.0; 95% CI 1.4–2.9).[22] The greatest mortality risk attributable to a hospital's low volume was noted for patients undergoing pancreatectomy (77.6%). National statistics have also been used to show similar findings for gastrectomy, oesophagectomy and liver lobectomy in Taiwan;[23] oesophagectomy and pancreatectomy in England;[24] oesophagectomy, pancreatectomy and hepatic resection in Scotland (Fig. 7.1);[25] and pancreatectomy in Italy.[26]

Length of Stay

In the same study by Hollenbeck, et al. as quoted above, prolonged hospitalisation was higher in LV centres compared with HV centres following oesophagectomy (11.3% vs. 5.2%; adjusted OR of prolonged hospitalisation 1.7; 95% CI 1.0–2.9) and pancreatectomy (13.7% vs. 7.8%; adjusted OR 1.6; 95% CI 1.2–2.2).[22] In another study of 38 hospitals between 1988 and 1993, the mean length of stay (LOS) following pancreatic resection was 23 days in Johns Hopkins Hospital compared with 27 days in LV hospitals throughout the rest of Maryland.[27] After laparoscopic gastrectomy, HV municipal or private-for-profit hospitals all exhibited shorter LOS and lower total costs compared with LV regional hospitals.[28]

Long-Term Survival

High hospital volume may not only be associated with reduced patient mortality in the immediate postoperative period but also with improved long-term survival. In one study of 2,592 pancreatic resections and 3,734 hepatic resections, HV centres (defined as >25 resections/year) demonstrated superior 5-year survival rates compared with LV centres, even after adjustment for demographics and comorbidities.[29] Using the

90 USA national Surveillance Epidemiology and End Results (SEER)-

Medicare linked database between 1992 and 2002, 5-year survival rates of upper GI cancer patients treated in HV centres was significantly higher compared with LV counterparts (oesophagectomy 34.0% vs. 17.0%; gastrectomy 32.0% vs. 25.6%; and pancreatectomy 15.9% vs. 10.8%). Interestingly, the use of postoperative adjuvant chemo/radiotherapy was reduced significantly in HV centres following oesophagectomy but was increased dramatically following pancreatectomy.[30] Other studies have also shown improved 5-year survival rates for patients with cancer of the oesophagus and gastric cardia in Swedish HV centres[31] and for patients undergoing hepatectomy for colorectal cancer metastases in NCI-designated cancer centres, and HV hospitals.[32]

Economic Cost

Interestingly, although some studies have shown reduced costs in HV centres,[27] this is not always the case. In Massachusetts between 1992 and 2000, the median cost for oesophagectomy was $755 greater in HV hospitals (NS), despite a two-day decrease in median LOS, a 3-day reduction in median ICU stay, an increased rate of home discharges (rather than rehabilitation) and a 3.7 fold decrease in hospital mortality.[33] There are, of course, many possible explanations for this in a primarily private health care system, which will not be explored further in this chapter.

Key Point

- Increased volume is associated with more accurate preoperative staging, superior quality of surgical resection, reduced postoperative morbidity and mortality, decreased length of stay, and improved long-term survival of upper GI cancer patients.

INDIVIDUAL SURGEON VOLUME AND UPPER GI CANCER SURGERY

Although not investigated as often as hospital volume, surgeon volume has been shown to be probably equally important in the determination of patient outcome. One study of liver resections (n=2949) from the USA demonstrated that when socioeconomic factors had been adjusted, hospital volume did not influence postoperative mortality unless the operation was performed by a HV surgeon in a HV centre.[34] However, yet other studies have suggested that LV surgeons operating within a HV unit with appropriate training can achieve good results for oesophagectomy.[35]

In a similar way to hospital volume, 'surgeon volume' can also be defined in a number of different ways, including individual surgeon caseload, sub-specialisation, completion of speciality training and experience. In the systematic review by Chowdhury, et al. 74 per cent of **91** surgeon caseload studies and 91 per cent of surgeon-speciality studies demonstrated a positive VOR.[11] However, some of the markers used to measure sub-specialisation or speciality training in these studies are quite soft, e.g. surgeon membership of specialty associations. No studies, to date, have analysed accumulated logbook experience as a measure of training or experience. Surgeon age has also been used as a surrogate measure of experience in some studies. When patients undergoing gastrectomy were operated on by surgeons aged over 50 years, they had a better 5-year survival rate compared to patients operated on by younger surgeons.[36] However, evidence also suggests that the relationship between surgeon age and patient outcome following complex surgical procedures might be U-shaped. Compared with surgeons aged 41 to 50 years, surgeons aged over 60 years had higher mortality rates following pancreatectomy (adjusted OR 1.67; 95% CI 1.12–2.49) but the detrimental effect of age was restricted largely to those surgeons with low procedure volumes.[37]

SPECIFIC AREAS WHERE SURGEON VOLUME INFLUENCES OUTCOME

Quality of Surgery

HV surgeons may offer more advanced operations unavailable to patients of LV surgeons. Evidence suggests that the Ivor-Lewis oesophagectomy provides improved 5-year survival for patients with type I junctional tumours and improved loco-regional disease-free survival for patients with one to eight lymph nodes, compared with other types of resection.[38] HV surgeons performed a greater number of Ivor-Lewis oesophagectomies compared with LV surgeons (95% vs. 73%, respectively, when HV defined as >6 cases/year)[39] and minimally invasive oesophagectomies.[40] Interestingly, in the latter study (which also demonstrated a reduced postoperative mortality rate for HV surgeons) the majority of HV surgeons (87%) practiced in an academic setting and had cardiothoracic training, whilst most LV surgeons were general surgeons in private practice (52.3%).[40]

Postoperative Mortality

In Canada, hepatobiliary subspecialty training has been shown to be predictive of the postoperative complication rate after hepatic resection,[41] whereas, in Japan, HV surgeons had fewer complications after total gastrectomy (n=136; morbidity rates 11% for HV surgeons vs. 24% for LV).[42]

Postoperative Complications

In one English study, the relative risk of postoperative mortality following
oesophagectomy was higher for LV surgeons (mean of 4 resections/year),

compared with HV surgeons (mean of 11 resections/year) (relative risk 4.6; mortality rate 17% vs. 4%), although there was no difference in subsequent long-term survival.[36] In south and west England, the 30-day mortality rate following oesophagectomy decreased by 40 per cent for every increase of 10 cases/year in surgeon volume compared with a decrease of only 8 per cent for every increase of 10 cases/year in hospital volume.[43] In comparison, the decreases in mortality rate following gastrectomy were 41 per cent and 7 per cent respectively.[43] Surgical training has also been shown to influence postoperative mortality. Surgeons trained in upper GI specialty surgery (defined as membership of the specialist society) had superior adjusted mortality rates following gastrectomy (6.5% vs. 8.7% for non-specialty trained surgeons; adjusted OR = 0.70; 95% CI 0.46–1.08) although this difference was not significant.[44] After adjustment for patient demographics, thoracic surgeons certified by the American Board of Thoracic Surgery had significantly lower adjusted mortality rates following oesophageal resection compared with non-specialist surgeons following oesophageal resection (12.5% vs. 16.5%; p<0.01).[45] However, the effect of training was diminished by incorporation of hospital volume in the analysis and was lost after accounting for surgeon volume. Therefore, both hospital and surgeon volume were more important predictors of outcome than subspecialty training.

Long-Term Survival

Following gastric cancer resection, patients of LV surgeons had worsened 6-month and 5-year survival rates (adjusted mortality hazard ratio 1.3 for LV surgeons compared with HV).[36] Higher surgeon volume was also predictive of better 5-year survival following hepatic resection for hepatocellular carcinoma (HCC) in Taiwan, whereas hospital volume was not significant.[46] Interestingly, survival rates of HCC patients were also influenced by physician volume as well as surgeon volume.[47]

Economic Cost

After adjustment for treatment and prognosis, costs per patient demonstrated a U-shaped relationship with doctor volume for patients with pancreatic, oesophageal and gastric cancer in the UK following presentation to hospital.[48] The authors concluded that the nature of this relationship reflected active interventions by HV doctors but long inpatient stays with little activity by LV doctors. Thus, intermediate volume (IV) doctors were associated with the lowest costs.

FACTORS UNDERLYING THE VOLUME-OUTCOME RELATIONSHIP

The factors that underlie the hospital VOR and surgeon VOR are complex but they are undoubtedly similar and overlap. The involvement of a multi-disciplinary team at all stages in the care pathway is crucial. Key determinants include preoperative staging and decision-making,[49] the role of neo-adjuvant chemo/radiotherapy,[50] intraoperative team skills, and critical care in the postoperative period.[51] There is no doubt that it remains difficult to separate the differential effects of the VOR from general improvements in surgical/anaesthetic and critical care skills over the past 20 to 30 years, during the time period when overall number of resections for upper GI cancer (except gastric cancer) has increased. However, when examined longitudinally, the increase in resections has tended to be in HV hospitals with numbers in LV hospitals falling sometimes to zero.[25] As an example of the general improvements in upper GI cancer care over time, it was shown that in a single Italian institution over the 25-year period between 1980 and 2004, an increasing proportion of oesophagectomy patients underwent neo-adjuvant chemotherapy and had earlier stage tumours in resected specimens, plus the R0 resection rate increased from 74.5 per cent to 90.1 per cent.[52] Below are highlighted specific examples of studies that highlight specific mechanistic factors underlying the VOR.

Preoperative Factors

Studies have shown that preoperative staging investigations may be more accurate in HV centres.[49]

Intraoperative Factors

Upper GI cancer resections are known to have a learning curve[53] and therefore, HV surgeon experience of the necessary operation augmented by subspecialty training provides the technical skills required for a successful operation and satisfactory patient outcome. Analysis of 150 consecutive Ivor-Lewis oesophagectomies performed by a single surgeon revealed consistent technical improvement over a 7-year period, including reduced single lung operating time, blood loss, transfusion requirement, ITU stay and LOS, and increased lymph node yield.[53] The presence of other expert surgical colleagues in a HV hospital may also allow opportunities for collaboration and operating together. Working regularly with HV anaesthetists/ICU staff not only provides patient cardiovascular stability and ensures adequate postoperative analgesia[51] but also allows the development of teamwork and structured protocols. In addition, HV centres may offer operations not available at LV hospitals (e.g. laparoscopic-assisted gastrectomy, which on meta-analysis, has been shown to have reduced blood loss and fewer complications compared with open distal gastrectomy for early gastric cancer).[54] Interestingly though, the presence of similar operations within a HV hospital has not demonstrated an impact on outcome following upper GI cancer resection.

For example, the presence of a liver transplant programme was not associated with improved 30-day mortality following hepatic resection.[55]

Postoperative Factors

Although adverse event rates appear to be similar between HV, IV and LV centres, the ability to 'rescue' these patients appears to be very different. The failure-to-rescue rate (mortality following an adverse event) following resection was only 0.7% in HV centres, which was less than one-fifth of that seen in the other centres,[56] suggesting that early recognition of problems (e.g. early endoscopy to detect gastric tube ischaemia following oeosphagectomy) followed by rapid and appropriate intervention is better in HV hospitals with more experienced staff. Following gastrectomy, a greater number of available critical care beds were associated with reduced postoperative mortality,[56] suggesting that infrastructure and available facilities are also important factors in patient outcome. There is also some evidence, albeit in benign upper GI disease that LV centres adhere less to guidelines (e.g. for cholecystectomy[57] and upper GI bleeding[58]) and management practice may vary between academic and non-academic doctors (e.g. acute peptic ulcer bleeding[59]), implying that the knowledge base of doctors working in LV centres might not be fully up-to-date.

Key Point

- Proposed mechanisms for the positive volume-outcome relationship include skills, experience and quality in the multi-disciplinary fields of preoperative patient selection, neo-adjuvant/adjuvant oncological therapy, specialist surgery, and postoperative care.

IMPORTANCE OF STUDY DESIGN

When judging the published literature on VORs, it is important to consider the impact that study methods might have on the findings. Furthermore, it should be noted that, to date, no randomised controlled trial has been performed to assess the role of hospital/surgeon volume on patient outcome following upper GI cancer resection.

Definition of Volume

For each type of surgical resection, there are no agreed definitions of what constitutes 'high' or 'low' volume and therefore, the use of volume cut-offs varies between studies. Some authors have employed arbitrary cut-offs based on expert opinion,[29] whereas others have used cut-offs based on percentiles.[25] Importantly, these cut-offs should be chosen before examining outcome data in order to avoid bias.

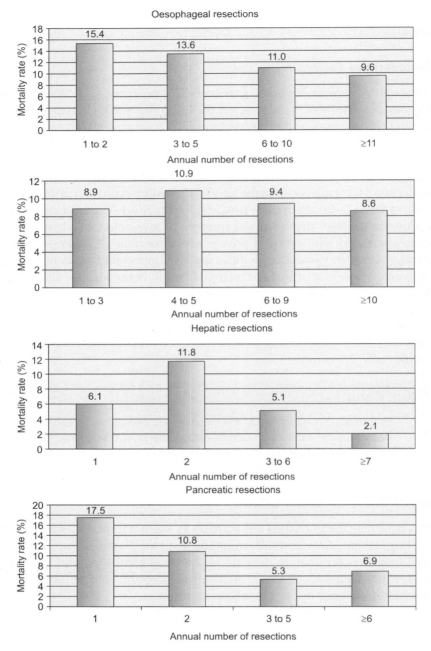

Fig. 7.1: Postoperative mortality rates for elective upper GI cancer resections according to quartile of hospital-year volume in Scotland 1982–2003. Adapted from Skipworth, et al. 2009. The mortality rates following oesophageal, hepatic and pancreatic resections increased as hospital-year volume increased. In this actual study, the data for gastric resections did not achieve statistical significance. a = statistically different from lowest volume quartile, p<0.01; b = statistically different from lowest volume quartile, p<0.001; c = statistically different from second volume quartile, p<0.01; d = statistically different from second volume quartile, p<0.001.

Data Source and Analysis

When considering procedural volume, different sources have been used to generate the data, including cancer registries, discharge summaries and estimates based on insurance claims. Such sources are known to be not 100% accurate, leading to misclassification of data.[60] Furthermore, some studies have relied on significant assumptions imposed upon the data source. As hospital and surgeon volumes are also likely to vary annually, questions remain as to how volume data should be analysed. Some studies have averaged data over several years to obtain mean volume,[10] whereas others have considered volume-years independently (Fig. 7.1).[25] In comparison, surgical specialty is most often considered as a dichotomous categorical variable but it can also be analysed as a continuous variable by considering procedural diversity. Using billing codes, procedural diversity can be analysed using the Herfindahl-Hirschman index, an economic concept that is a measure of the size of firms in relation to the overall industry,[61] although results may be influenced by how broadly or narrowly specialisation is defined.

Adjustment for Case-mix

The results of VOR studies can only be used as reliable performance indicators if they are accompanied by case-mix information.[62] It is possible that some LV hospitals may be more likely to admit patients with comorbidities and to be from poorer socio-economic and ethnic backgrounds.[10] Furthermore, LV hospitals may receive higher rates of non-elective admissions compared with HV centres depending on geography. Data from colorectal cancer studies have shown a reduced risk of perioperative death for HV surgeons when performing elective but not emergency surgery.[63] Thus, adjustment of data to account for such confounding factors is essential. Some authors have attempted to stratify quantitatively patient risk by using scoring systems such as the Physiological and Operative Severity Score for the enuUmeration of Mortality and Morbidity [POSSUM]) to avoid such bias.[64]

In one systematic review of the cancer VOR literature (n=272 papers reviewed and 135 included covering 27 procedures and clinical conditions), studies were most commonly excluded because volume was not an independent variable (n=43) or samples were not population-based (n=40). Risk adjustments were performed most frequently using administrative data (60%) and clinical data (28%; although only 10 studies [7%] were considered to be robustly discriminating and well-calibrated), whereas 12% had no risk adjustment. Only five studies adjusted for the type of resection or the use of adjuvant therapy.[65] In another meta-analysis (n=101 articles reporting 137 cancer studies), common methodological limitations were failure to control for confounders, post hoc categorisation of provider volume and unit of analysis errors.[66]

Key Point

- The findings of volume outcome studies may be influenced by both the data source and the method of statistical analysis. No randomised control trials of high volume providers versus low volume providers have been reported.

EFFECT OF THE VOLUME-OUTCOME RELATIONSHIP ON SERVICE PROVISION

It is now generally accepted that both hospital and surgeon volume have a significant influence on patient outcome in upper GI cancer surgery (Fig. 7.2). This recognition has in turn driven a major reorganisation of surgical services in the UK[67] and other countries.

Centralisation of Surgical Services

Regionalisation and centralisation of upper GI cancer surgery has taken place gradually over the last decade or so in many countries but has undoubtedly accelerated recently.[25,68] This has, not surprisingly, had a major effect on LV hospitals. However, improvements in patient outcome will remain the main driver for change. Centralisation in the Cologne and Bonn regions of Germany (as a result of VOR-based regulations) resulted in 34 per cent of hospitals stopping oesophageal surgery and 8 per cent stopping pancreatic surgery.[69] In the Netherlands, centralisation was associated with a decrease in postoperative mortality following oesophagectomy from 12 per cent to 4 per cent, with related reductions in postoperative morbidity and LOS.[70] Regionalisation of pancreatic cancer surgery in Ontario, Canada, resulted in improved mortality over a 10-year period (10.4% to 2.2%), with the percentage of operations performed in HV centres increasing from 33 per cent to 71 per cent.[71] In Maryland, USA, centralisation of pancreatic resections was attributed as the single most important cause of the reduction in postoperative mortality from 17.2 per cent in 1984 to 4.9 per cent in 1995.[72] An estimated 61 per cent of the decline in the mortality rate was attributable to the increase in caseload at the HV provider. In countries reliant on private healthcare systems, such centralisation initiatives are supported by industry. In the USA, the Leapfrog Group, a consortium of Fortune 500 corporations and healthcare purchasers harnesses their purchasing power to improve the quality of care via the regionalisation of complex surgical procedures in high volume centres.[73]

Quality Improvement Strategies

The concept of 'exporting surgical excellence' or adopting recognised protocols for safe surgery has led to improved patient outcomes in both LV centres[73] and academic institutions.[74] Following published evidence of a positive VOR for pancreatic cancer resections in Ontario, a province-level quality improvement strategy prompted some surgeons to discontinue operating, although many surgeons had concerns regarding the number of cases required to be considered HV.[75] Simple attempts at standardisation of surgical training and practice can also yield successful results. Following the Dutch D1/D2 gastric cancer trial (1989–1993), the 5-year patient survival rates were shown to improve.[76]

Recommended Ideal Volume Thresholds

Positive VOR studies have led some authors to estimate the theoretical number of lives that might be saved by moving patients from LV centres to HV ones. In a meta-analysis of VOR cancer studies (n=101 articles reporting 137 studies), the effect of doubling case volume on the OR of mortality was 0.81 for oesophagectomy (95% CI 0.77–0.84), 0.88 for gastrectomy (95% CI 0.86–0.91), 0.77 for liver resection (95% CI 0.72–0.83) and 0.78 for pancreatectomy (95% CI 0.73-0.84).[66] The number of patients that needed to be moved from a hospital in the lower volume quartile to a hospital in the upper volume quartile to prevent one volume-associated death was therefore calculated as: oesophagectomy 10, gastrectomy 50, liver resection 11 and pancreatectomy 13. These calculations were obviously dependent on the study definition of volume but authors have also concluded that the annual number of lives saved by moving operations from local LV to HV centres could be as much as four per year for oesophagectomy and six per year for pancreaticoduodenectomy.[77]

One might assume that the most obvious conclusion following evidence of a positive VOR would be the proposal of recommended volume thresholds for upper GI cancer centres and surgeons. Using national Scottish data, it has been estimated that surgical units must perform at least 51 oesophagectomies, 41 gastrectomies, 24 hepatectomies and 33 pancreatectomies per year to ensure average mortality rates of less than 5%.[25] Other authors have suggested that a hospital should perform more than 20 oesophagectomies per year to ensure mortality rates less than 10%.[78] A recent report by the Association of Upper GI Surgeons of Great Britain and Ireland (AUGIS) has recommended that the ideal oesophago-gastric unit should consist of four to six surgeons each carrying out a minimum of 15 to 20 resections per year, serving a population of 1–2 million.[79] In comparison, the ideal hepato-biliary unit should consist of a team of six surgeons each carrying out a minimum of 12 to 16 pancreatic resections per year and 15 to 25 liver resections (10–15 major) per year, serving a population of 2 to 3 million. However, because of differences in case-mix and geography, several authors have concluded that it is never possible to identify a unique volume threshold.[80] Others have claimed that volume is an imperfect surrogate of quality of care and that it is insufficient for defining centres of excellence alone.[66,81,82] This notion is supported by data that the suggested volume may only explain less than 1% of variance in perioperative death.[82]

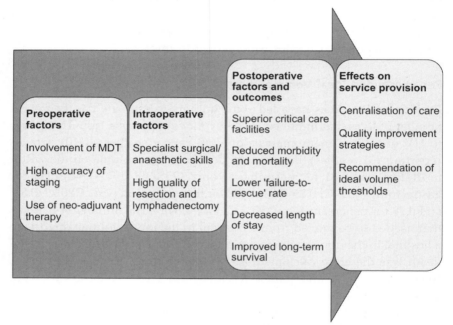

Fig. 7.2: The process of the volume-outcome relationship in resectional surgery for upper GI cancer. The figure demonstrates the pre-, intra- and postoperative factors hypothesised to be the cause of the positive volume-outcome relationship, the superior patient outcomes that result from the relationship and the subsequent effects on service provision that the relationship drives.

Key Point

- The positive volume-outcome relationship has led, in many countries, to the centralisation of upper GI cancer services, the development of strategies to export surgical quality to low volume centres and the publication of recommended ideal volume thresholds.

CONCLUSIONS

On the balance of evidence, both hospital and surgeon volume are major determinants of patient outcome following upper GI cancer resections.

Not surprisingly this has led to the centralisation of surgical services in many countries, perhaps at the expense of increased costs and the unfortunate discontinuation of some LV centres with previously good results. However, with changes to surgical training and the reduction in working hours now evident across most of Europe, and progressively worldwide, it is likely that this process of centralisation will continue. This in turn is likely to see further improvements in patient outcome while at the same time underpinning subspecialty training and support for the next generation of upper GI surgeons.

Key Points For Clinical Practice

- Many studies have suggested that hospital volume and surgeon volume are both key determinants of outcome following oesophageal, gastric, pancreatic and liver resections
- It is unclear as to whether hospital volume or surgeon volume is the more important determinant of outcome
- Increased volume is associated with more accurate preoperative staging, superior quality of surgical resection, reduced postoperative morbidity and mortality, decreased length of stay, and improved long-term survival of upper gastrointestinal (GI) cancer patients
- Proposed mechanisms for the positive volume-outcome relationship include skills, experience and quality in the multi-disciplinary fields of preoperative patient selection, neo-adjuvant/adjuvant oncological therapy, specialist surgery and postoperative care
- The findings of volume outcome studies may be influenced by both the data source and the method of statistical analysis. No randomised control trials of high volume providers versus low volume providers have been reported
- The positive volume-outcome relationship has led, in many countries, to the centralisation of upper GI cancer services, the development of strategies to export surgical quality to low volume centres and the publication of recommended ideal volume thresholds.

REFERENCES

1. Hannan EL, Radzyner M, Rubin D, et al. The influence of hospital and surgeon volume on in-hospital mortality for colectomy, gastrectomy, and lung lobectomy in patients with cancer. Surgery. 2002;131(1):6-15.
2. Begg CB, Cramer LD, Hoskins WJ, et al. Impact of hospital volume on operative mortality for major cancer surgery. JAMA. 1998;280(20):1747-51.
3. Hannan EL, Racz M, Kavey RE, et al. Pediatric cardiac surgery: The effect of hospital and surgeon volume on in-hospital mortality. Pediatrics. 1998;101(6):963-9.
4. Holt PJ, Poloniecki JD, Loftus IM, et al. Meta-analysis and systematic review of the relationship between hospital volume and outcome following carotid endarterectomy. Eur J Vasc Endovasc Surg. 2007; 33 (6):645-51.

5. Holt PJ, Poloniecki JD, Gerrard D, et al. Meta-analysis and systematic review of the relationship between volume and outcome in abdominal aortic aneurysm surgery. Br J Surg. 2007;94(4):395-403.

6. Ananthakrishnan AN, McGinley EL, Saeian K. Higher hospital volume is associated with lower mortality in acute nonvariceal upper-GI hemorrhage. Gastrointest Endosc. 2009;70(3):422-32.

7. Nguyen NT, Paya M, Stevens CM, et al. The relationship between hospital volume and outcome in bariatric surgery at academic medical centers. Ann Surg. 2004;240(4):586-93.

8. Safford SD, Pietrobon R, Safford KM, et al. A study of 11,003 patients with hypertrophic pyloric stenosis and the association between surgeon and hospital volume and outcomes. J Pediatr Surg. 2005;40(6):967-72.

9. Patti MG, Corvera CU, Glasgow RE, et al. A hospital's annual rate of esophagectomy influences the operative mortality rate. J Gastrointest Surg. 1998;2(2):186-92.

10. Birkmeyer JD, Siewers AE, Finlayson EV, et al. Hospital volume and surgical mortality in the United States. N Engl J Med. 2002;346(15):1128-37.

11. Chowdhury MM, Dagash H, Pierro A. A systematic review of the impact of volume of surgery and specialization on patient outcome. Br J Surg. 2007;94(2):145-61.

12. Killeen SD, O'Sullivan MJ, Coffey JC, et al. Provider volume and outcomes for oncological procedures. Br J Surg. 2005;92(4):389-402.

13. Verhoef C, van de Weyer R, Schaapveld M, et al. Better survival in patients with esophageal cancer after surgical treatment in university hospitals: a plea for performance by surgical oncologists. Ann Surg Oncol. 2007;14(5):1678-87.

14. Birkmeyer NJ, Goodney PP, Stukel TA, et al. Do cancer centers designated by the National Cancer Institute have better surgical outcomes? Cancer. 2005;103(3):435-41.

15. Dimick JB, Cowan JA Jr, Colletti LM, et al. Hospital teaching status and outcomes of complex surgical procedures in the United States. Arch Surg. 2004;139(2):137-41.

16. van Vliet EP, Eijkemans MJ, Kuipers EJ, et al. A comparison between low-volume referring regional centers and a high-volume referral center in quality of preoperative metastasis detection in esophageal carcinoma. Am J Gastroenterol. 2006;101(2):234-42.

17. Bilimoria KY, Talamonti MS, Wayne JD, et al. Effect of hospital type and volume on lymph node evaluation for gastric and pancreatic cancer. Arch Surg. 2008;143(7):671-8.

18. Reid-Lombardo KM, Gay G, Patel-Parekh L, et al. Treatment of gastric adenocarcinoma may differ among hospital types in the United States, a report from the National Cancer Data Base. J Gastrointest Surg. 2007;11(4):410-9.

19. Bilimoria KY, Talamonti MS, Sener SF, et al. Effect of hospital volume on margin status after pancreaticoduodenectomy for cancer. J Am Coll Surg. 2008;207(4):510-9.

20. Dimick JB, Pronovost PJ, Cowan JA, et al. Surgical volume and quality of care for esophageal resection: do high-volume hospitals have fewer complications? Ann Thorac Surg. 2003;75(2):337-41.

21. Reavis KM, Smith BR, Hinojosa MW, et al. Outcomes of esophagectomy at academic centers: an association between volume and outcome. Am Surg. 2008;74(10):939-43.

22. Hollenbeck BK, Dunn RL, Miller DC, et al. Volume-based referral for cancer surgery: informing the debate. J Clin Oncol. 2007;25(1):91-6.

23. Lin HC, Xirasagar S, Lee HC, et al. Hospital volume and inpatient mortality after cancer-related gastrointestinal resections: the experience of an Asian country. Ann Surg Oncol. 2006;13(9):1182-8.

24. Pal N, Axisa B, Yusof S, et al. Volume and outcome for major upper GI surgery in England. J Gastrointest Surg. 2008;12(2):353-7.

25. Skipworth RJ, Parks RW, Stephens NA, et al. The relationship between hospital volume and postoperative mortality rates for upper gastrointestinal cancer resections: Scotland 1982-2003. Eur J Surg Oncol. 2010;36(2):141-7.

26. Balzano G, Zerbi A, Capretti G, et al. Effect of hospital volume on outcome of pancreaticoduodenectomy in Italy. Br J Surg. 2008;95(3):357-62.

27. Gordon TA, Burleyson GP, Tielsch JM, et al. The effects of regionalization on cost and outcome for one general high-risk surgical procedure. Ann Surg. 1995;221(1):43-9.

28. Kuwabara K, Matsuda S, Fushimi K, et al. Effect of hospital charateristics on the quality of laparoscopic gastrectomy in Japan. Gastroenterol Res. 2010;3(2):65-73.

29. Fong Y, Gonen M, Rubin D, et al. Long-term survival is superior after resection for cancer in high-volume centers. Ann Surg. 2005;242(4):540-4.

30. Birkmeyer JD, Sun Y, Wong SL, et al. Hospital volume and late survival after cancer surgery. Ann Surg. 2007;245(5):777-83.

31. Wenner J, Zilling T, Bladstrom A, et al. The influence of surgical volume on hospital mortality and 5-year survival for carcinoma of the oesophagus and gastric cardia. Anticancer Res. 2005;25(1B):419-24.

32. Wang X, Hershman DL, Abrams JA, et al. Predictors of survival after hepatic resection among patients with colorectal liver metastasis. Br J Cancer. 2007;97(12):1606-12.

33. Kuo EY, Chang Y, Wright CD. Impact of hospital volume on clinical and economic outcomes for esophagectomy. Ann Thorac Surg. 2001;72(4):1118-24.

34. Eppsteiner RW, Csikesz NG, Simons JP, et al. High volume and outcome after liver resection: surgeon or center. J Gastrointest Surg. 2008;12(10):1709-16.

35. Jeganathan R, Kinnear H, Campbell J, et al. A surgeon's case volume of oesophagectomy for cancer does not influence patient outcome in a high volume hospital. Interact Cardiovasc Thorac Surg. 2009;9(1):66-9.

36. Xirasagar S, Lien YC, Lin HC, et al. Procedure volume of gastric cancer resections versus 5-year survival. Eur J Surg Oncol. 2008;34(1):23-9.

37. Waljee JF, Greenfield LJ, Dimick JB, et al. Surgeon age and operative mortality in the United States. Ann Surg. 2006;244(3):353-62.

38. Omloo JM, Lagarde SM, Hulscher JB, et al. Extended transthoracic resection compared with limited transhiatal resection for adenocarcinoma of the mid/distal esophagus: five-year survival of a randomized clinical trial. Ann Surg. 2007;246(6):992-1000.

39. Migliore M, Choong CK, Lim E, et al. A surgeon's case volume of oesophagectomy for cancer strongly influences the operative mortality rate. Eur J Cardiothorac Surg. 2007;32(2):375-80.

40. Enestvedt CK, Perry KA, Kim C, et al. Trends in the management of esophageal carcinoma based on provider volume: treatment practices of 618 esophageal surgeons. Dis Esophagus. 2010;23(2):136-44.

41. McKay A, You I, Bigam D, et al. Impact of surgeon training on outcomes after resective hepatic surgery. Ann Surg Oncol. 2008;15(5):1348-55.

42. Fujita T, Yamazaki Y. Influence of surgeon's volume on early outcome after total gastrectomy. Eur J Surg. 2002;168(10):535-8.

43. Bachmann MO, Alderson D, Edwards D, et al. Cohort study in South and West England of the influence of specialization on the management and outcome of patients with oesophageal and gastric cancers. Br J Surg. 2002;89(7):914-22.

44. Callahan MA, Christos PJ, Gold HT, et al. Influence of surgical subspecialty training on in-hospital mortality for gastrectomy and colectomy patients. Ann Surg. 2003;238(4):629-36.

45. Dimick JB, Goodney PP, Orringer MB, et al. Specialty training and mortality after esophageal cancer resection. Ann Thorac Surg. 2005;80(1):282-6.

46. Lin HC, Lin CC. Surgeon volume is predictive of 5-year survival in patients with hepatocellular carcinoma after resection: a population-based study. J Gastrointest Surg. 2009;13(12):2284-91.

47. Chen TM, Chang TM, Huang PT, et al. Management and patient survival in hepatocellular carcinoma: does the physician's level of experience matter? J Gastroenterol Hepatol. 2008;23(7 Pt 2):e179-88.

48. Bachmann M, Peters T, Harvey I. Costs and concentration of cancer care: evidence for pancreatic, oesophageal and gastric cancers in National Health Service hospitals. J Health Serv Res Policy. 2003;8(2):75-82.

49. Davies AR, Deans DA, Penman I, et al. The multidisciplinary team meeting improves staging accuracy and treatment selection for gastro-esophageal cancer. Dis Esophagus. 2006;19(6):496-503.

50. Allum WH, Stenning SP, Bancewicz J, et al Long-term results of a randomized trial of surgery with or without preoperative chemotherapy in esophageal cancer. J Clin Oncol. 2009;27(30):5062-7.

51. Robertson SA, Skipworth RJ, Clarke DL, et al. Ventilatory and intensive care requirements following oesophageal resection. Ann R Coll Surg Engl. 2006;88(4):354-7.

52. Ruol A, Castoro C, Portale G, et al. Trends in management and prognosis for esophageal cancer surgery: twenty-five years of experience at a single institution. Arch Surg. 2009;144(3):247-54.

53. Sutton DN, Wayman J, Griffin SM. Learning curve for oesophageal cancer surgery. Br J Surg. 1998;85(10):1399-402.

54. Ohtani H, Tamamori Y, Noguchi K, et al. Meta-analysis of Laparoscopy-Assisted and Open Distal Gastrectomy for Gastric Cancer. J Surg Res. 2010.

55. Dixon E, Schneeweiss S, Pasieka JL, et al. Mortality following liver resection in US medicare patients: does the presence of a liver transplant program affect outcome? J Surg Oncol. 2007;95(3):194-200.

56. Smith DL, Elting LS, Learn PA, et al. Factors influencing the volume-outcome relationship in gastrectomies: a population-based study. Ann Surg Oncol. 2007;14(6):1846-52.

57. Nguyen GC, Boudreau H, Jagannath SB. Hospital volume as a predictor for undergoing cholecystectomy after admission for acute biliary pancreatitis. Pancreas. 2010;39(1):e42-7.

58. Maiss J, Schwab D, Ludwig A, et al. Medical and endoscopic treatment in peptic ulcer bleeding: a national German survey. Z Gastroenterol 2010;48(2):246-55.

59. Cheung J, Sawisky G, Enns R, et al. Practices in peptic ulcer bleeding controversies among university- versus nonuniversity-affiliated gastroenterologists. Can J Gastroenterol. 2010;24(4):261-5.

60. Hollenbeck BK, Hong J, Zaojun Y, et al. Misclassification of hospital volume with Surveillance, Epidemiology, and End Results Medicare data. Surg Innov. 2007;14(3):192-8.

61. Hall BL, Hsiao EY, Majercik S, et al. The impact of surgeon specialization on patient mortality: examination of a continuous Herfindahl-Hirschman index. Ann Surg. 2009;249(5):708-16.

62. Wouters MW, Wijnhoven BP, Karim-Kos HE, et al. High-volume versus low-volume for esophageal resections for cancer: the essential role of case-mix adjustments based on clinical data. Ann Surg Oncol. 2008;15(1):80-7.

63. Borowski DW, Kelly SB, Bradburn DM, et al. Impact of surgeon volume and specialization on short-term outcomes in colorectal cancer surgery. Br J Surg. 2007;94(7):880-9.

64. Sah BK, Zhu ZG, Chen MM, et al. Effect of surgical work volume on postoperative complication: superiority of specialized center in gastric cancer treatment. Langenbecks Arch Surg. 2009;394(1):41-7.

65. Halm EA, Lee C, Chassin MR. Is volume related to outcome in health care? A systematic review and methodologic critique of the literature. Ann Intern Med. 2002;137(6):511-20.

66. Gruen RL, Pitt V, Green S, et al. The effect of provider case volume on cancer mortality: systematic review and meta-analysis. CA Cancer J Clin. 2009;59(3):192-211.

67. National Cancer Guidance Steering Group/Cancer Guidance Group of the Clinical Outcomes Group. Guidance on Commissioning Cancer Services: Improving Outcomes in Upper Gastro-intestinal Cancers—The Manual. London: Department of Health 2001.

68. Al-Sarira AA, David G, Willmott S, et al. Oesophagectomy practice and outcomes in England. Br J Surg. 2007;94(5):585-91.

69. Roeder N, Wenke A, Heumann M, et al. [Volume-outcome relationship. Consequences of reallocation of minimum volume based on current German surgical regulations]. Chirurg. 2007;78(11):1018-27.

70. Wouters MW, Karim-Kos HE, le Cessie S, et al. Centralization of esopha-geal cancer surgery: does it improve clinical outcome? Ann Surg Oncol. 2009;16(7):1789-98.

71. Simunovic M, Urbach D, Major D, et al. Assessing the volume-outcome hypothesis and region-level quality improvement interventions: pancreas cancer surgery in two Canadian Provinces. Ann Surg Oncol. 2010;17(10):2537-44.

72. Gordon TA, Bowman HM, Tielsch JM, et al. Statewide regionalization of pancreaticoduodenectomy and its effect on in-hospital mortality. Ann Surg. 1998;228(1):71-8.

73. Maa J, Gosnell JE, Gibbs VC, et al. Exporting excellence for Whipple resection to refine the Leapfrog Initiative. J Surg Res. 2007;138(2):189-97.

74. Kennedy EP, Grenda TR, Sauter PK, et al. Implementation of a critical pathway for distal pancreatectomy at an academic institution. J Gastrointest Surg. 2009;13(5):938-44.

75. Wright FC, Fitch M, Coates AJ, et al. A Qualitative Assessment of a Provincial Quality Improvement Strategy for Pancreatic Cancer Surgery. Ann Surg Oncol. 2010 [Epub ahead of print].

76. Krijnen P, den Dulk M, Meershoek-Klein Kranenbarg E, et al. Improved survival after resectable non-cardia gastric cancer in The Netherlands: the importance of surgical training and quality control. Eur J Surg Oncol. 2009;35(7):715-20.

77. Urbach DR, Bell CM, Austin PC. Differences in operative mortality between high- and low-volume hospitals in Ontario for 5 major surgical procedures: estimating the number of lives potentially saved through regionalization. CMAJ. 2003;168(11):1409-14.

78. Metzger R, Bollschweiler E, Vallbohmer D, et al. High volume centers for esophagectomy: what is the number needed to achieve low postoperative mortality? Dis Esophagus. 2004;17(4):310-4.

79. Association of Upper Gastrointestinal Surgeons. (2011). AUGIS Reports. [online] AUGIS website. Available from http://www.augis.org/news_guidelines/augis_reports.htm [Accessed January 2011]

80. Davoli M, Amato L, Minozzi S, et al. [Volume and health outcomes: an overview of systematic reviews]. Epidemiol Prev. 2005;29(3-4 Suppl):3-63.

81. Gasper WJ, Glidden DV, Jin C, et al. Has recognition of the relationship between mortality rates and hospital volume for major cancer surgery in California made a difference?: A follow-up analysis of another decade. Ann Surg. 2009;250(3):472-83.

82. Meguid RA, Weiss ES, Chang DC, et al. The effect of volume on esophageal cancer resections: what constitutes acceptable resection volumes for centers of excellence? J Thorac Cardiovasc Surg. 2009; 137(1):23-9.

SECTION THREE

LOWER GASTROINTESTINAL TRACT

CHAPTER EIGHT

Modern Management of an Intestinal Fistula

Sturt NJH, Windsor ACJ, Engledow AH

INTRODUCTION

An intestinal or enterocutaneous fistula (ECF) is an abnormal communication between the mucosal epithelium of the intestinal tract and another epithelial surface. In the majority of clinical contexts this second epithelial surface is the skin of the abdominal wall (Fig. 8.1) and this review will focus on the modern management of such ECF.

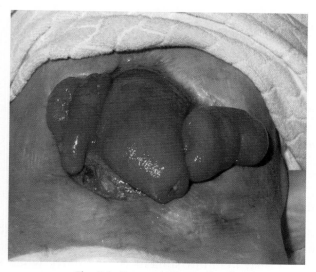

Fig. 8.1: Enterocutaneous fistula

AETIOLOGY

In the majority of cases intestinal fistulae are the result of the complications arising after abdominal surgery. In a small minority of cases fistulae arise spontaneously as a consequence of other pathologies such as Crohn's disease, malignancy or radiotherapy, but such fistulae represent a small proportion of the overall fistula workload. In postoperative fistulae the usual underlying mechanism is either disruption of a surgical anastomosis or inadvertent enterotomy with subsequent leakage of intestinal content through the surgical incision in the abdominal wall.

Key Point

- The majority of enterocutaneous fistulae arise as a consequence of the complications of abdominal surgery.

RISK FACTORS AND THE PREVENTION OF FISTULATION

Risk factors for the development of fistula following abdominal surgery may be divided into preoperative, perioperative and postoperative factors. A summary of these risk factors is shown in Table 8.1.

TABLE 8.1

List of factors predisposing to the development of enterocutaneous fistula

Preoperative
- Previous abdominal surgery
- Malnourishment
- Operations for inflammatory bowel disease
- Active sepsis
- Steroid use
- Intra-abdominal abscess/fistula

Perioperative
- Shocked/septic patient
- Extensive adhesiolysis
- Injudicious anastomoses

Postoperative
- Repeat laparotomy

Preoperative Risk Factors (correcting what is reversible)

Preoperative risk factors predisposing to ECF formation include operations for inflammatory bowel disease, presence of previous abdominal surgery, malnourishment (particularly when the serum albumin is less than 30 g/L), active sepsis, steroid use (e.g. more than 10 mg prednisolone per day), the presence of an intra-abdominal abscess and the presence of a pre-existing antral fistula. For example, looking at the latter, four risk factors in the context of surgery for Crohn's disease, Yamamoto et al. found a ten-fold increase in the risk of postoperative abscess, fistula or anastomotic leak in patients with all four risk factors compared with those patients with none (5% compared with 50% risk).[1]

This being the case it is mandatory to pre-optimise patients as far as possible prior to surgery to reduce such risk factors. This would include treating sepsis and abscesses pharmacologically and radiologically, optimising nutrition and weaning steroids to a minimum. When it is not possible to pre-optimise patients, (particularly in the emergency setting) serious consideration should be given to the use of stomas and the avoidance of anastomoses altogether (as given below).

Perioperative Risk Factors, Surgical Decision Making and the Judicious Use of Stomas

Postoperative ECF usually arise as a result of disrupted anastomoses or inadvertent enterotomy sustained during adhesiolysis. Thus meticulous surgical technique and repair of inadvertent enterotomy or serosal tears during surgery is very important, especially in preoperative surgery. Likewise, judgement needs to be exercised in determining whether an anastomosis should be fashioned or whether a stoma brought out. In our unit, we try to avoid anastomoses in malnourished patients (particularly those with serum albumin less than 20 g/L), septic patients, patients who are shocked, patients on substantive doses of steroids and in situations where an anastomosis will lie in a pre-existing abscess cavity. It is important to remember that a high-output, high jejunostomy will be easier to manage than a high-output ECF.

Postoperative Risk Factors: Avoidance of Repeat Laparotomies

It goes without saying that postoperative complications will be minimised by careful management of fluid balance, nutrition, early mobilisation and so forth. The most important postoperative consideration however is the avoidance of repeat laparotomies unless absolutely necessary.

The rate of inadvertent enterotomy in repeat laparotomies increases in a near linear relationship depending on the number of prior operations. Van der Krabben et al. showed that patients with three or more previous laparotomies had an odds ratio of 10.4 (95% CI:5.0–21.6) of sustaining enterotomy during surgery compared with those patients with fewer previous operations.[2] The risk is particularly great during the so-called 'window of doom' occurring between 10 days and 6 weeks following initial surgery when immature adhesions cause the abdomen to be particularly hostile and therefore prone to iatrogenic injury. Therefore, before embarking on reoperative surgery for the management of complication (particularly more than 10 days postoperatively), it is very important to question whether further surgery is really necessary, or whether the complication could be managed in a different way, for example with radiological drainage of abscesses.

Key Points

- Prevention is much better than cure and the risks can be lessened by pre-optimisation of patients, meticulous surgical technique, the judicious sue of stomas and careful postoperative management
- Re-laparotomy following abdominal surgery is arguably the greatest risk factor for the development of a fistula and should only be undertaken if a clear indication is present

POORLY MANAGED SURGICAL CATASTROPHE

No matter how meticulous the surgery, surgical catastrophes will inevitably happen. The critical aspect is how it is dealt with when it occurs.

Clinical Course of a Poorly Managed Intestinal Fistula

Typically patients will not do well following initiating abdominal surgery and may suffer a prolonged ileus and unexplained sepsis. There is then likely to be a partial or even complete dehiscence of their abdominal wound which may initially discharge pus, but over time begins to discharge intestinal content. This bowel content damages the surrounding skin whilst undrained intra-abdominal collections cause episodes of sepsis and promote the overall catabolic state. Loss of electrolytes, predominantly sodium, and water, lead to electrolyte imbalances, dehydration and worsen the patient's clinical condition further. Inabilities to absorb sufficient nutrients combined with the catabolic state worsen the patient's nutritional status and contribute further to their overall decline. An inexperienced surgeon may then attempt to 'fix the problem' surgically during the early stages when adhesions are at their most severe, and patients at their most septic, malnourished and unwell. This leads to further inadvertent bowel injury and a completely unclosable abdomen with multiple uncontrolled fistulae and a worse situation than before. In the face of such management mortality of fistulae is high.

When Repeat Laparotomy is Mandatory

Despite the great importance of avoiding unnecessary re-operation in the early postoperative period there do exist some definitive indications for re-operation following the complications of abdominal surgery and these are shown in Table 8.2. The surgical principles in such a situation are to do as limited a procedure as possible.

TABLE 8.2

List of indications for re-laparotomy in the early postoperative period

- Generalised peritonitis
- Deterioration despite radiological drainage
- Multiple/septate collections not drainable radiologically
- Ischaemic bowel
- Abdominal compartment syndrome/worsening intra-abdominal hypertension
- Inability to protect the skin from intestinal content.

Principles to be Followed in Complicated Cases

- Repair, i.e. control the source of infection. Practically speaking in most cases this would involve the construction of a stoma proximal to an anastomotic leak or fistula, or taking down a leaking anastomosis and bringing both ends out as a double-ended stoma.
- Purge thorough peritoneal toilet
- Prevention and control of recurrent infection (again, generally by proximal diversion of intestinal content) and debridement of dead tissue
- Treatment of intra-abdominal hypertension. This involves a high index of suspicion, measurement of transvesical pressures and serious consideration of leaving the abdomen open as a laparostomy (often with a vacuum-assisted dressing) with planned closure in the future

A complete guide to management of the open abdomen lies outside the scope of this chapter, however, it is worth noting that without careful management the natural history of an open abdomen is of the worsening from a clean wound without fascia adherence or lateral fixity towards the more severe grades involving fixity (frozen abdomen) and fistulation.[3]

OCCURRENCE OF FISTULA

When fistulation has occurred, meticulous management is critical in dictating the subsequent outcome for the patient. The main principles of control of sepsis, provision of adequate nutrition and fluid balance and then planned repair are summed by the acronyms SNAPP (Sepsis, Nutrition, Anatomy of the fistula, Protection of the skin and Planned procedure), or SOWATS (Sepsis, Optimise nutrition, wound care, Anatomy, Timing of surgery and Strategy of surgery).[4] Each of the components of the SOWATS acronym will now be examined in turn.

Sepsis

Of all the aspects of fistula management, sepsis is the most important, with an early review of the treatment of ECF showing that 65% of deaths attributable to ECFs were directly related to sepsis.[5] The same paper showed that in patients where sepsis was not adequately controlled the mortality was 85%. It therefore cannot be overemphasised how important it is that sepsis be aggressively managed right from the outset. In series from St Mark's and UCH Hospitals, 75% of deaths in ECF patients were directly attributable to sepsis.[6,7]

The principles of sepsis management revolve around judicious use of broad-spectrum antibiotics with adequate coverage of gut organisms, and early CT scanning of patients displaying signs of sepsis such as spiking temperatures, rising inflammatory markers and clinical deterioration despite adequate nutritional support. Antibiotic therapy may be guided by culture results and it is important to consider infection with fungal organisms, particularly in debilitated patients. Intra-abdominal collections should be drained radiologically wherever possible with many patients requiring repeated interventional procedures. Only in the context of factors shown in Table 8.2 should sepsis be treated by surgical re-intervention.

Key Points

- Sepsis is the major cause of mortality in patients with intestinal fistula and should be managed aggressively, preferably with radiological drainage and antibiotics.
- Initial management consists of eradication of sepsis, optimisation of fluid balance, nutrition and protection of the skin. Some fistulae are likely to close spontaneously, those that do not will require surgical repair.

Wound Care

Intestinal content is corrosive due to the presence of proteolytic enzymes, and left unchecked, it will severely damage the skin around the fistula. It is obviously therefore very important that the skin is protected, generally using a wound manager (Fig. 8.2). Early and continued involvement of stoma therapists is indicated to ensure the skin remains protected. Use of a vacuum dressing where the fistula is isolated has been tried but is specialised and labour intensive, so is probably best confined to specific situations where the necessary expertise is available. Failure to protect the skin around an ECF is one of the indications for early surgical reintervention.

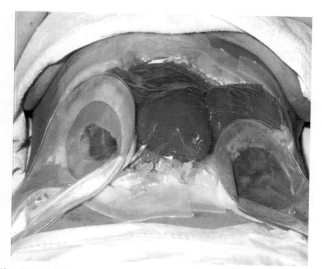

Fig. 8.2: Fistula seen in the previous figure following application of wound manager and appropriate skin protection

Nutrition

For the purposes of simplicity, management of fluid and electrolyte balance will be considered together with nutrition in this section.

Physiology

Under normal circumstances the upper gastrointestinal tract secretes around 7 litres of fluid into the lumen of the bowel in a 24 hour period, the great majority of which is absorbed in the distal small bowel and colon. In the proximal jejunum sodium and water enter the lumen of the gut prior to absorption more distally. Where there is a proximal small bowel fistula or high jejunostomy (and thus no downstream absorption), the presence of hypotonic fluid in the proximal jejunum will exacerbate both sodium and water excretion into the lumen and worsen sodium and water depletion. Conversely the presence of hypertonic, sodium rich fluid will encourage sodium and water absorption and decrease loss.

Fluid Balanc—Working out the Basal Output

It is well determined that fistulas with a low basal output have a better chance of spontaneous closure than those with a higher output. Since output is dependent on oral intake, an initial period of nil by mouth for 48 hours in the absence of pharmacological agents which affect output will help to establish the fistula basal output. During this time patients' fluid, electrolyte and nutritional needs are managed parenterally. Those patients with an output more than 1 litre/24 hours are very unlikely to undergo spontaneous fistula closure, will almost certainly need parenteral nutrition (PN) and plans can be made accordingly. In those patients with output less than 500 ml/24 hours there is a high chance of spontaneous closure and patients are unlikely to require PN. Patients with an intermediate (500–1000 ml/24 hours) have a less certain clinical course and it is worth attempting to control output to bring about reduction and possibly decrease the need for PN and increase the chance of spontaneous closure.

Decreasing Output

Reducing fistula output both reduce fluid, electrolyte and nutrient loss and may also increase the chance of spontaneous closure. Use a step by step regimen with the next step being added on, if the preceding one does not give a satisfactory reduction in output.

Step 1: Appropriate Isotonics and Fluid Restriction

The traditional mantra of encouraging patients to drink lots of hypotonic fluids to counteract excessive output actually has the opposite effect due to the reasons explained above. For this reason patients should be restricted to a total of 1500 ml/24 hours orally. A litre of this should be oral electrolyte solution such as St Mark's solution or double-strength dioralyte™ solution (i.e. 10 sachets/litre of water). Fruit cordials may be added to improve palatability. The remaining 500 ml of fluid can be of the patient's choice. Drinking should be discouraged within 30 minutes of meals.

Step 2: Proton Pump Inhibition

Proton pump inhibitors decrease output by decreasing gastric secretion. Doses of 40–80 mg omeprazole every 24 hours are appropriate.

Step 3: Loperamide and Codeine Phosphate

Loperamide is a very useful drug for decreasing output, and it is safe, even at large doses. A typical starting dose would be 4 mg QDS, but this can be increased up to at least 16 mg QDS to increase effect. Codeine may further reduce output and doses of up to 60 mg QDS may be used.

Step 4: Octreotide

Octreotide is a somatostatin analogue which has been shown to decrease both pancreatic and small bowel fluid secretion. Its use in small bowel fistulas is controversial with evidence from 11 small studies showing limited evidence of benefit.[8] It is reasonable to commence therapy at a dose of 200 micrograms subcutaneously TDS for 48 hours. If after 48 hours there has been no benefit (e.g. a reduction in output of more than 300 ml/ 24 hours) then the agent should be stopped as there is no evidence that it will subsequently make any difference to the outcome.

High Output Despite Intervention

If after instituting the above measures output remains above 1 litres/ 24 hours then it is exceedingly unlikely that the fistula will close spontaneously, and also certain that the patient will require parenteral support. Patients should be allowed to eat normally as desired. Unless home parenteral support can be arranged the patient may need to stay in hospital until definitive surgery is performed.

Low Output

Those patients with an output less than 500 ml/24 hours have a good chance of spontaneous closure and rarely require parenteral support. Such patients may be allowed to have a normal diet and be feed up for early discharge.

Intermediate Group

The intermediate group is more of a challenge as output may be critical in dictating spontaneous closure. Every effort should therefore be made to decrease output to a minimum and there is a possible case for total parenteral nutrition with nil by mouth, although this is contentious.

Monitoring Fluid and Electrolyte Status

Patients should have daily blood tests to monitor electrolyte levels including magnesium. Overall body sodium levels are better measured with urinary sodium than with blood levels. The aim is a well hydrated patient with fistula output less than 1500 ml/24 hours, more than 1 litre urine output/24 hours, urinary sodium more than 20 mmol/litre, serum magnesium more than 0.7 mmol/litre and body weight within 10% of normal.

Nutrition

Patients require the input of an experienced dietician. Many patients will require at least a period of parenteral nutrition, and many will require high protein oral supplements. The aim is for stable or rising albumin without continuing weight loss.

ANATOMY—THE CHANCE OF SPONTANEOUS CLOSURE AND APPROPRIATE INVESTIGATIONS

In terms of planning, it is important to estimate the chance of spontaneous fistula closure. Table 8.3 shows the factors which determine the likelihood of a fistula closing spontaneously. Four studies have shown a spontaneous closure rate of up to 30%.[6,9-11] Another older study showed that 90% of those fistulas which closed spontaneously did so within the first month, with the remaining 10% occurring within the next two months, and none thereafter.[5] Thus, if a fistula has not closed within three months it is exceedingly unlikely to do so.

Appropriate investigations to determine anatomy include CT scanning with oral contrast, small bowel follow-through studies and fistulograms. The relevant questions being required of the investigation are to define the anatomy (i.e. site of fistula, anatomy of the tract and the residual small bowel anatomy), and to determine if there is any downstream discontinuity or obstruction.

TABLE 8.3

Factors influencing the likelihood of spontaneous closure of enterocutaneous fistula

	Favourable	Not favourable
Output	Low (<500 ml/24 hours)	High (>1000 ml/24 hours)
Anatomy of fistula tract	Long and narrow	Short and wide
Small bowel	No active disease No distal obstruction No mucocutaneous continuity No intestinal discontinuity	Active disease Distal obstruction Mucocutaneous continuity Intestinal discontinuity
Patient	Previously fit and well	Significant co-morbidity

Timing of Surgery—More Art than Science

A study in 2004 showed that the longer the delay between the onset of fistulation and attempted repair, the less the recurrence rate.[11] Patients operated on within 2–12 weeks of their initial operation had a 28% chance of recurrence compared with a rate of 15% in those whose operation was carried out more than 12 weeks following fistula formation. It thus seems mandatory to wait at least six weeks following fistula formation if at all possible. Traditional dogma dictated waiting six months between the onset of a fistula and attempted surgical repair. A more modern approach is a so-called physiological approach, since some patients may be optimised

TABLE 8.4:

Factors determining readiness for surgical repair of enterocutaneous fistula

Physiological

- Sepsis adequately treated
- Nutritionally replete/ positive nitrogen balance

Abdominal hostility

- Abdomen soft, clinical lack of induration
- Granulating woundProlapsing bowel loops

Time since fistula development

- Minimum 6 weeks
- Usual time around 6 months

Psychology

- Patient psychologically ready/prepared

for surgery before this six month period, whilst others may require a longer time.

Table 8.4 shows the parameters used to determine when surgery should be considered when planning operation for intestinal fistula. Assessment of abdominal hostility is largely a clinical exercise, with a hard, woody abdomen indicating underlying hostility, whilst a soft, compliant abdomen suggests that the underlying adhesions are soft and operable.

Key Points

- Planning surgery involves determining the anatomy of the tract and remaining bowel
- Timing of surgery is very important and depends on a number of factors, many of them determined by clinical assessment. The usual minimum is to wait six weeks since fistula onset, but a more usual time frame would be six months
- Surgery involves resection of the fistula rather than attempted repair. Anastomoses are minimised and stomas constructed if there is significant doubt about the safety of anastomoses

STRATEGY OF SURGERY

The ultimate goals of surgery are restoration of intestinal continuity (either by anastomosis or via the route of temporary or permanent stoma) and reconstruction of the inevitable abdominal wall defect.

Dealing with the Fistula

The skin to either side of the fistula is incised and the abdominal wall is separated from the underlying adhesions (Fig. 8.3). The entire small bowel is then meticulously dissected from the proximal landmark of the

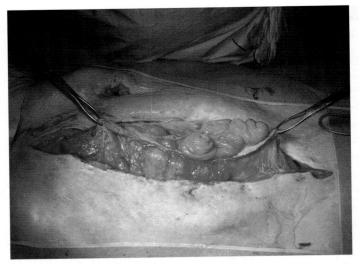

Fig. 8.3: Dissection of fistula away from underlying abdominal wall prior to resection and abdominal wall reconstruction

duodenojejunal (DJ) flexure to the distal landmark of the ileocaecal valve. Care is taken to prevent inadvertent enterotomy, with any serosal injuries being oversewn. The fistula itself is resected rather than an attempt being made to repair the defect. A proximal stoma may be fashioned or if felt safe, an anastomosis. The principle of minimising anastomoses is followed and anastomoses are avoided altogether if the rules of safe anastomosis are going to be breached.

Reconstructing the Abdominal Wall

It is inevitable that there is going to be an abdominal wall defect once the fistula is repaired. After such a long period of time there is near-inevitable lateral fixity of the fascia of the abdominal wall.

One strategy is primary closure. For small defects this may be readily achievable and it has the advantage of avoidance of implanting prosthetic material into the abdomen with the potential risks which this involves.

Achieving lateral closure may be more difficult when there is a larger defect and excessive lateral fixity. Here, the component separation technique of Ramirez can be useful to achieve a tension-free closure.[12] In this technique, the superficial abdominal wall is separated from the underlying fascia to a point just lateral to the linea semilunaris (i.e. the point at which the anterior rectus sheath ends and the aponeurosis of the external oblique begins). The medial edge of the externus aponeurosis is then incised along its length, cranial to caudal, and the layer is dissected off the underlying internal oblique muscle. In the original description, the medial edge of the posterior rectus sheath is also incised and separated from the muscle although this step seems optional and is difficult where the hernial defect has distorted the anatomy of the medial part of the abdominal wall.

Use of the component separation technique can achieve and extra 10 cm or so on each side to make primary closure achievable.

Use of Prosthetic Mesh

A review of long-term follow-up after incisional hernia repair showed that recurrence rates were almost halved by the use of mesh compared with primary repair.[13] The use of mesh therefore seems attractive in repairing the defect in the abdominal wall, and in cases where primary closure is not possible even with component separation, its use would seem mandatory.

The key problem with this in the context of enterocutaneous fistula is that, by definition, the operative field is contaminated by the fistula, so that traditional non-absorbent prosthetic mesh is highly likely to become infected after placement.

The traditional means of dealing with this is by a two-staged approach. Here, either a defect is deliberately left at the end of a procedure, or a temporary absorbable mesh such as vicryl™ is used to create a temporary repair with the expectation that a new hernia will inevitably occur. Once the infection and operative field have settled down fully, a second planned procedure is carried out using a non-absorbable mesh with definitive hernia repair. Whilst being a valid approach, this does commit the patient to further surgery with the additional expense and morbidity which this poses.

Use of Biological Mesh

The use of decellularised collagen matrices (either allograft or xenograft) is now well established in the field of incisional hernia repair. The principle theoretical advantages of biological mesh are that it becomes incorporated into the scar by means of cellular in-growth into the matrix (resulting in a robust repair) and that in theory it is resistant to infection. Biological mesh may be used as an inlay repair, as an onlay (i.e. as an adjunct to primary closure) or as an inlay bridge when full defect closure is not possible. The principle disadvantage of biological mesh is that it is far more expensive than the equivalent non-biological prosthesis, although this expense may be offset if it allows a one-stage as opposed to a two-stage repair.

In this unit, the authors have recently presented (in abstract form) their experience of using the non cross-linked porcine-derived biological mesh Strattice™ in a series of 24 contaminated ventral hernias (Windsor, AC, personal communication). In a median follow-up of five months there was one hernia recurrence and no mesh infections.

Superficial abdominal wall dehiscence over the mesh occurred in a number of patients; however, this was managed with vacuum-assisted dressings or simple packing without further problems. Biological meshes would therefore seem a highly valid technique for abdominal wall reconstruction following enterocutaneous fistula repair, although the results of published, peer reviewed studies are awaited.

Key Point

- Repair of the abdominal wall defect is a key part of the procedure. If primary closure cannot be achieved an absorbable mesh may be used and a later definitive repair planned. More recently the use of biological mesh has enabled one-stage repair even in a contaminated field

FOLLOW-UP FOLLOWING ENTEROCUTANEOUS FISTULA REPAIR

Recurrence rates following ECF repair are approximately 15%.[4-7] Of those with recurrence in one recent series from the author's institution, three-quarters healed spontaneously without the need for further surgery.[7]

Rehabilitation following these long and critical illnesses should not be forgotten. Rarely if ever do these patients go back to living a completely normal life. Many will require subsequent surgical intervention for ongoing complications. Many will have significant bowel function changes. In addition, some will end up with short bowel syndrome and on long term home parenteral feeding. It is also worth pointing out that in addition to the obvious physical insult these patients are often psychologically very traumatised by these events and may require additional input in the often long and difficult recovery phase. There often remains reluctance to return to their original referring hospital and so long journeys to the regional centre and the logistics of that are also not to be underestimated.

CONCLUSION

Intestinal fistula is usually the result of surgical complications. The outcome for the patient is largely determined by the quality of the subsequent management. With optimal management, the outlook for the patient is good with low mortality and recurrence of fistula.

Key Points for Clinical Practice

- The majority of enterocutaneous fistulae arise as a consequence of the complications of abdominal surgery
- Prevention is much better than cure and the risks can be lessened by pre-optimisation of patients, meticulous surgical technique, the judicious sue of stomas and careful postoperative management

- Re-laparotomy following abdominal surgery is arguably the greatest risk factor for the development of a fistula and should only be undertaken if a clear indication is present
- Sepsis is the major cause of mortality in patients with intestinal fistula and should be managed aggressively, preferably with radiological drainage and antibiotics
- Initial management consists of eradication of sepsis, optimisation of fluid balance and nutrition and protection of the skin. Some fistulae are likely to close spontaneously, those that do not will require surgical repair
- Planning surgery involves determining the anatomy of the tract and remaining boweltiming of surgery is very important and depends on a number of factors, many of them determined by clinical assessment. The usual minimum is to wait six weeks since fistula onset, but a more usual time frame would be six months
- Surgery involves resection of the fistula rather than attempted repair. Anastomoses are minimised and stomas constructed if there is significant doubt about the safety of anastomoses. Repair of the abdominal wall defect is a key part of the procedure. If primary closure cannot be achieved an absorbable mesh may be used and a later definitive repair planned. More recently the use of biological mesh has enabled one-stage repair even in a contaminated field

REFERENCES

1. Yamamoto T, Allan RN, Keighley MR. Risk factors for intra-abdominal sepsis after surgery in Crohn's disease. Dis Colon Rectum 2000;43(8):1141-5.
2. Van Der Krabben AA, Dijkstra FR, Nieuwenhuijzen M, et al. Morbidity and mortality of inadvertent enterotomy during adhesiotomy. Br J Surg 2000;87(4):467-71.
3. Bjorck M, Bruhin A, Cheatham M, et al. Classification-important step to improve management of patients with an open abdomen. World J Surg 2009;33(6):1154-7.
4. Visschers RG, Olde Damink SW, Winkens B, et al. Treatment strategies in 135 consecutive patients with enterocutaneous fistulas. World J Surg 2008;32(3):445-53.
5. Reber HA, Roberts C, Way LW, et al. Management of external gastrointestinal fistulas. Ann Surg 1978;188(4):460-7.
6. Hollington P, Mawdsley J, Lim W, et al. An 11-year experience of enterocutaneous fistula. Br J Surg 2004;91(12):1646-51.
7. Datta V, Engledow A, Chan S, et al. The management of enterocutaneous fistula in a regional unit in the United Kingdom: a prospective study. Dis Colon Rectum 2010;53(2):192-9.
8. Lloyd DA, Gabe SM, Windsor AC. Nutrition and management of enterocutaneous fistula. Br J Surg 2006;93(9):1045-55.

9. Campos AC, Meguid MM, Coelho JC. Factors influencing outcome in patients with gastrointestinal fistula. Surg Clin North Am 1996;76(5):1191-8.

10. Li J, Ren J, Zhu W, et al. Management of enterocutaneous fistulas: 30-year clinical experience. Chin Med J (Engl). 2003;116(2):171-5.

11. Lynch AC, Delaney CP, Senagore AJ, et al. Clinical outcome and factors predictive of recurrence after enterocutaneous fistula surgery. Ann Surg 2004;240(5):825-31.

12. Ramirez OM. Abdominal herniorrhaphy. Plast Reconstr Surg 1994;93(3):660-1.

13. Burger JW, Luijendijk RW, Hop WC, et al. Long-term follow-up of a randomized controlled trial of suture versus mesh repair of incisional hernia. Ann Surg 2004;240(4):578-83.

CHAPTER■ NINE

Rectal and Pelvic Prolapse

Dirk Weimann, David Jayne

INTRODUCTION

The last decade has seen increasing interest in the surgical treatment of pelvic organ prolapse. Much of this has been technology driven with the introduction of laparoscopic techniques and new stapling devices. This has been accompanied by a better understanding of the pathophysiology, and in particular the recognition that internal rectal prolapse is an anatomical entity worthy of surgical repair. The concept of rectal and pelvic organ prolapse has thus evolved with novel methods aimed at correcting the anatomical defects and restoring normal physiological function. There is better appreciation that rectal and other pelvic organ prolapses are seldom isolated pathological conditions, but rather they are often symptomatic of a global pelvic floor failure. Multidisciplinary teams involving coloproctologists, urogynaecologists, urologists, radiologists, physiotherapists and other allied health professionals, are increasing recognised as the preferred means for providing speciality care for this complex group of patients. Thus, there has been an incremental shift in clinical practise, which is continuing to evolve.

This chapter aims to provide an overview of current thinking in rectal and pelvic organ prolapse with particular emphasis on newer surgical techniques. The entirety of pelvic organ prolapse cannot be adequately covered in a single chapter, and therefore priority is given to posterior compartment failure, namely full-thickness rectal prolapse and internal rectal prolapse. For the avoidance of confusion, the terms internal rectal prolapse and intussusception will be used synonymously.

FULL-THICKNESS RECTAL PROLAPSE

Full-thickness rectal prolapse refers to protrusion of the complete rectal tube through the anal canal. Clinically it needs to be distinguished from muco-haemorrhoidal prolapse, in which protrusion of the distal anorectal mucosa occurs only.

Full-thickness rectal prolapse is a distressing condition where the patient is aware of a lump emerging from the anus, which may or may not reduce spontaneously. It is more common in females than males by a factor of 10 to 1 with the incidence in females increasing with advancing age;[1] a feature which is not apparent in males.[2] Bleeding, ulceration, and mucous discharge, due to repeated trauma are frequent complaints. There is usually anorectal discomfort, but pain is infrequent unless the prolapse is irreducible with developing ischaemia. Invariably, there is a degree of anal sphincter weakness which may manifest as either faecal leakage or incontinence depending on the degree of sphincter dysfunction and associated constipation. Assessment of incontinence and constipation is important, as they have a bearing on the surgical approach.

The aetiology of full-thickness prolapse is unclear. In few cases there may be a link with collagenous connective tissue disorders, but for the majority the precipitating cause is not obvious. Its occurrence is associated with a deep pouch of Douglas, laxity of the pelvic floor, weak sphincter muscles with or without pudendal neuropathy, and lack of normal fixation of the rectum.

Imaging of the colon and rectum, with flexible sigmoidoscopy as a minimum, is mandatory to exclude a prolapsing neoplasm or other co-existent pathology. It is the authors' practice to undertake anorectal manometry and endoanal ultrasound on all patients with rectal prolapse prior to proceeding to surgery to establish baseline sphincter function, although it is accepted that this is not universal practice. Proctography is of limited value in full-thickness prolapse with its use restricted to the few cases where there is diagnostic uncertainty or difficulty in distinguishing full-thickness from internal rectal prolapse or muco-haemorrhoidal prolapse. If slow transit constipation is suspected, then colonic marker studies may be useful and, if supportive a resectional rectopexy may be preferred.

Choice of Surgical Procedure

Conventional teaching advocates an abdominal approach in medically fit patients, due to lower rates of recurrent prolapse, with perineal approaches reserved for patients with significant co-morbidity. The widespread introduction of laparoscopic techniques challenges this ideology, with the elderly and frail being more readily able to tolerate a laparoscopic abdominal repair than a conventional open procedure. Resectional rectopexy is usually recommended for those patients who suffer slow transit constipation with the caveat that there is a morbidity and even mortality associated with the anastomosis.

Abdominal Procedures

Posterior Rectopexy

The benefits of the laparoscopic approach are evident following posterior rectopexy, although this does not exclude an open approach if necessary.[3] A variety of methods are described which differ in the extent of rectal mobilisation, the method of rectal fixation, and whether performed in combination with a resection. Controversy exists as to whether the lateral ligaments, if they are present as a distinct entity, should be divided or left *in situ*. The argument for taking the ligaments is that it allows for better resuspension with less recurrence, whilst the counter-argument is that division may contribute to rectal denervation and increased postoperative constipation.[4,5] A variety of fixation methods are described including suture fixation to the sacral promontory, use of a posterior mesh, and laparoscopic tacking of the lateral ligaments to the sacrum. Mesh should probably be avoided in favour of sutured fixation if rectopexy is combined with sigmoid resection to minimise infective complications.

The recurrence rate following posterior rectopexy is usually low (< 5%). Interpretation of the data regarding postoperative constipation is difficult due to heterogeneity of studies and surgical technique. Following laparoscopic rectopexy postoperative constipation has been reported in around 70 per cent of patients,[6,7] although improved constipation has also been reported in 41 per cent of patients.[8] Generally, incontinence is improved in 50 to 80 per cent of patients,[6-10] although several months may be necessary to allow for anal sphincter recovery.

Resectional Rectopexy

Resectional rectopexy is usually reserved for those patients with full-thickness prolapse and documented slow transit constipation. The rectopexy part of the operation proceeds as for posterior rectopexy; with the exception that suture fixation to the sacral promontory is usually preferred in the presence of an anastomosis. A sigmoid colectomy is combined with the rectopexy in anticipation that it will remove redundant colon and lessen postoperative constipation.[4]

Ventral Rectopexy

Ventral rectopexy is gaining popularity on the basis that it avoids posterior rectal dissection and hence better preserves autonomic innervation, which in turns helps to reduce postoperative constipation.[11] The procedure is well suited to a laparoscopic approach and can be undertaken with short lengths of hospital stay and an early return to normal activities. The procedure involves suturing of a strip of mesh into the rectovaginal (rectoprostatic in males) septum with fixation of the mesh at the sacral promontory. The main concerns with this approach centre on long-term mesh complications.[12]

The technique will be described further in treatment options for internal rectal prolapse (as given below).

Perineal Procedures

Delorme's Procedure

Probably the most straightforward and still most widely used of the perineal operations: the Delorme's procedure involves a muscular plication of the rectal tube to invaginate and fix the prolapse. At operation, a circumferential incision is made through the mucosa of the prolapsed rectum at 1 to 2 cm from the dentate line. The mucosal lining is dissected off the underlying muscular tube to just beyond the apex of the prolapse. The dissected mucosa is excised and the muscular tube plicated with a series of longitudinally orientated absorbable sutures, effectively reducing the prolapse. Mucosal apposition is secured with interrupted absorbable sutures.

Although a relatively straightforward and well tolerated operation, with mortality rates of 0 to 4 per cent,[13-15] the big drawback with the Delorme's procedure is the high rate of recurrent prolapse, which is variously reported between 4 to 27 per cent.[15,16] There is a general improvement in both constipation and incontinence.

Altemeier's Rectosigmoidectomy

A full-thickness circumferential incision is made through the outer layer of bowel wall involved in the prolapse. Anteriorly, the lower extent of the pouch of Douglas may be entered and care must be taken to avoid injury to any involved bladder. Rectosigmoidectomy proceeds with ligation of the mesorectum and contained vessels in close proximity to the bowel wall. The divided mesorectum is best suture ligated to prevent inadvertent slippage of ligatures, which may not be accessible through the transanal access. Resection continues cranially with progressive prolapse of the rectum until such point as the entire prolapsing bowel is delivered, which may involve some considerable length. The prolapsing bowel is amputated and a low colo-rectal anastomosis fashioned by either a hand-sewn or stapled technique.

The benefits claimed for Altemeier's operation over the Delorme's procedure include reduced rates of recurrent prolapse, with reported rates between 0 to 16 per cent.[17-19] Although a low anastomosis is involved, this does not appear to add to the mortality with reported rates of less than 5 per cent. The low anastomosis may, however, have an impact on functional outcomes with symptoms akin to anterior resection syndrome following low anterior resection.

Stapled Transanal Rectal Resection (STARR)

Stapled transanal rectal resection is usually reserved for patients with internal rectal prolapse. However, recent reports have indicated that the Transtar method for STARR can provide a safe and effective solution for lesser degrees of full-thickness rectal prolapse,[20,21] at least in the short-term. As such, STARR may have a role in those cases in which a Delorme's procedure is difficult due to the small size of the prolapse and where the prolapse is insufficient for an Altemeier's procedure. The Transtar stapler is a curved stapling device which enables the surgeon to undertake a circumferential full-thickness transanal rectal resection. When applied to full-thickness prolapse, the procedure in effect produces a stapled amputation of the prolapsing rectum. Short-term results in small series of patients suggest that it is a quick and effective procedure with associated improvements in incontinence.

Internal Rectal Prolapse

Internal rectal prolapse refers to invagination of the distal rectal wall into the rectal lumen during the course of straining to defaecate. Various grading systems have been proposed, which attempt to correlate the degree of prolapse with symptoms. Amongst these is the Oxford grading system which proposes the following classification:[22]

Grade 1: High rectorectal intussusception
Grade 2: Low rectorectal intussusception
Grade 3: High rectoanal intussusception
Grade 4: Low rectoanal intussusception
Grade 5: External rectal prolapse

Previous attempts at surgical repair of internal rectal prolapse by means of transanal repair,[23] rectopexy,[24] and anterior resection have met with variable success and as a consequence have not found popularity. However, in the last decade enthusiasm has been rekindled.

The clinical relevance of internal rectal prolapse is in its association with obstructed defecation. This syndrome may be defined as the normal desire to defecate but an inability to satisfactorily evacuate the rectum.

It consists of one or more of the following symptoms:
- Excessive straining to defecate
- Prolonged time spent on the toilet with fragmented defecation
- Incomplete evacuation with frequent returns to the toilet
- Dependency on laxatives and enemas
- Need for perineal support or digitation to initiate evacuation
- Occasional fresh rectal bleeding
- Anorectal discomfort.

Obstructed defecation may be functional in that there is no demonstrable anatomical abnormality, or mechanical in which case there is usually associated internal rectal prolapse with or without rectocele, enterocele or other pelvic organ prolapse. In the mechanical form, it is the internal prolapse descending and "plugging" the anal canal during straining which is believed to impede rectal evacuation (Fig. 9.1). Resolution of the internal prolapse and any associated rectocele with restoration of a more normal rectal anatomy is the aim of surgical repair.

Obstructed defecation is a common condition and should be discriminated from slow transit constipation by careful history, examination, and appropriate investigation. It is most frequently seen in middle-aged, multiparous women, but can occur in the nulliparous and even in males.

Investigation of suspected obstructed defecation is aimed at demonstrating a structural abnormality of the distal rectum which is amenable to surgical correction. Endoscopic assessment of the colorectum is mandatory to exclude co-existent pathology, but the mainstay of investigation is radiological imaging either in the form of dynamic

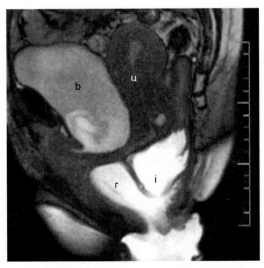

Fig. 9.1: MR proctography showing internal rectal prolapse (i), rectocoele (r), bladder (b), and uterus (u). Descent of the internal prolapse during defaecation "plugs" the anal canal and prevents satisfactory rectal evacuation.

proctography or magnetic resonance imaging (MRI). The author's preference is for proctographic imaging in cases of isolated posterior compartment (rectal) prolapse, with MRI reserved for multi-compartment symptomatology. The routine use of anorectal manometry and endoanal ultrasound is recommended because of the frequent association with faecal incontinence, which may be occult in the presence of over-riding constipation. Colonic marker studies may be helpful in detecting slow transit constipation.

Key Points

- Obstructed defecation is the normal desire to defecate, but an inability to satisfactorily evacuate the rectum. It is common in multiparous women.
- Both laparoscopic ventral rectopexy and STARR appear to be safe and effective in the treatment of obstructed defecation associated with internal rectal prolapse.
- Appropriate investigation and patient selection is paramount to successful outcomes when undertaking surgery for internal rectal prolapse.

Choice of Surgical Procedure

Internal Delorme's Procedure

This procedure may be considered as either a transanal version of the Delorme's operation for full-thickness rectal prolapse or a circumferential version of the Sarle's procedure for rectocoele repair.[25] A distal rectal mucosal flap is raised from just above the dentate line extending cranially for 5 to 8 cm. The underlying muscularis is plicated longitudinally with a series of absorbable sutures, excess mucosal flap is excised, and mucosa re-anastomosed to the dentate line, effectively obliterating the internal prolapse and any associated rectocoele. The procedure may be undertaken segmentally, which in combination produces a circumferential repair.

Although success with this technique has been claimed by some authors,[23,26] but in reality it is often a difficult and bloody procedure, and as a consequence it has failed to gain popularity.

Laparoscopic Sacrocolporectopexy (Ventral Rectopexy)

Ventral suspension for full-thickness rectal prolapse was first proposed by Ripstein in 1952.[27] In this procedure, the rectum is fully mobilised and fixed to the sacral promontory with an anterior sling of fascia lata or synthetic material. Although there is a trend to improvement in incontinence, mixed results are obtained in terms of constipation. With the introduction of laparoscopic techniques, the procedure was modified to limit posterior dissection of the rectum and minimise autonomic denervation.[12] The indication for laparoscopic ventral rectopexy was

131

subsequently extended to internal rectal prolapse for obstructed defaecation.[22,28,29]

The procedure involves a resuspension of the prolapsing distal rectum and any associated rectocele or enterocoele using a prosthetic mesh (Figs 9.2A to F). The right para-rectal gutter is dissected from the sacral promontory and extended across the anterior peritoneal reflection of the pouch of Douglas opening up the rectovaginal septum (rectoprostatic in the male). The rectovaginal septum is dissected as far as the pelvic floor and a strip of mesh sutured to the anterior rectal wall and the posterior vaginal vault. The mesh is put under tension and sutured or tacked to the bony sacral promontory, in effect providing resuspension and support to the posterior and middle pelvic floor compartments. The peritoneum is reconstituted in an attempt to minimise adhesive small bowel

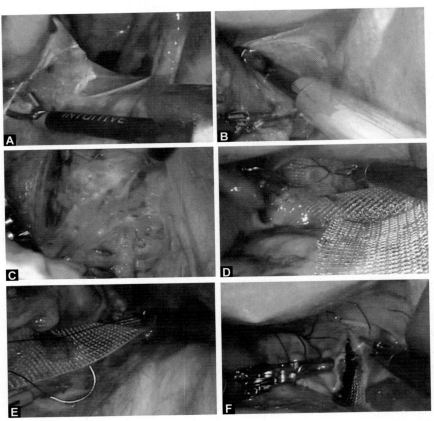

Figs 9.2A to F: Laparoscopic ventral rectopexy: (A) the peritoneum is opened at the sacral promontory; (B) and the incision extended down the right para-rectal gutter and across the anterior peritoneal reflection at the pouch of Douglas. (C) The rectovaginal septum is dissected to the level of the pelvic floor; (D) and a strip of mesh sutured to the anterior rectal wall and posterior vaginal vault. (E) The mesh is placed under tension and fixed to the sacral promontory. (F) The operation is completed by suture reconstitution of the peritoneum.

complications. If necessary, a "Y" shaped mesh can be used to provide simultaneous support to the anterior vaginal vault and bladder.

The results of laparoscopic ventral rectopexy for internal rectal prolapse are difficult to decipher due to heterogeneity in patient selection and operative technique. Short-term results suggest an improvement in both incontinence and constipation[28] and avoidance of posterior rectal mobilisation appears to protect against new onset evacuatory problems.[11]

Stapled Transanal Rectal Resection (STARR) and Transtar

Stapled transanal rectal resection was first described by Antonio Longo based on observations following stapled haemorrhoidopexy in patients with obstructed defaecation and internal rectal prolapse.[30]

It is proposed that excessive straining at defecation leads to laxity and thinning of the distal rectum, which in turn results in internal rectal prolapse and obstructed defaecation. Transanal resection of the prolapse together with any associated abnormality (rectocoele and mucohaemorrhoidal prolapse) was therefore advocated to correct the anatomy and restore normal evacuatory function. In addition, distal rectal resection results in a "-pexy" which at least partially corrects any perineal descent.

Due to the lack of a dedicated stapling device, STARR was originally described using two firings of a procedure for prolapse and haemorrhoids-01 (PPH-01) stapler (PPH, Ethicon Endosurgery, Cincinnati, USA). Subsequently, a specially designed curved stapling device became available, the Contour30 Transtar. Thus, at present there are two techniques for STARR; the PPH-STARR and Transtar. Both techniques produce a similar end result, namely a full-thickness, circumferential resection of the distal rectum together with any internal prolapse and rectocele.

In PPH-STARR, the prolapsing distal rectum is resected as separate anterior and posterior specimens, using two PPH-01 staplers (Figs 9.3A to D). In the Transtar technique the internal prolapse is resected with sequential firings of the Contour30 stapler (Figs 9.4A to D). The advantages claimed for Transtar include an ability to tailor the extent of resection, as there is no stapler housing to limit the amount of tissue to be resected, better visualisation of the resection, and a lack of the lateral "dog-ears" inherent in the PPH-01 method. Whether a tailored resection and lack of lateral "dog-ears" results in improved outcomes is debatable, with current evidence seeming to suggest this may not be the case.[31]

The evidence in support of STARR is increasing, with reports of several personal series, randomised trials,[32,33] and a large European Registry.[34] Initial concerns regarding safety, and in particular the risk of septic complications and rectovaginal fistulation, have not been borne out in the larger studies. Overall morbidity is in the region of 30 per cent, which includes all minor and major complications. The most frequently observed

133

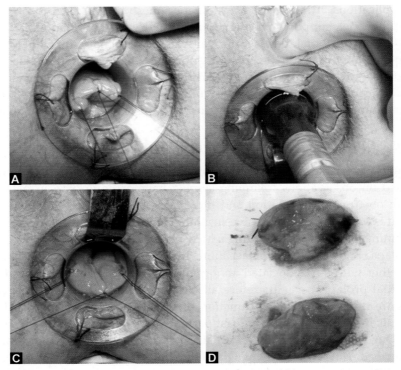

Figs 9.3A to D: PPH-STARR: (A) the anterior prolapse is held by 3 traction sutures. (B) The first of two PPH-01 staplers is inserted and used to perform a semi-circumferential anterior resection. The rectovaginal septum is checked to ensure it had not been incorporated in the stapler prior to firing. (C) The procedure is repeated for the posterior component of the prolapse with a second PPH-01 stapler. In both (B) and (C) a metal spatula is used to protect the opposite rectal wall from inadvertent inclusion in the stapler. (D) The two separate full-thickness resection specimens are shown

complications include anorectal pain (7.1%), urinary retention (6.9%), bleeding (5%), septic events (4.4%), and staple line complications (3.5%).[34] The current evidence suggests a short-term efficacy in the region of 80 per cent, with significant improvements in obstructed defaecation scores and health-related quality of life. However, concern has been expressed regarding the rate of postoperative defecatory urgency, which can affect up to 30 per cent of patients postoperatively, at least on a temporary basis. A reasonable proportion of these patients will have suffered urgency and poor sphincter function preoperatively, although some instances of de novo urgency are also apparent. With appropriate patient investigation and selection it should be possible to minimise this unwanted occurrence.[35]

Express Procedure

Originally developed as an alternative to the Delorme's procedure for full-thickness rectal prolapse,[36] the indications for the external pelvic

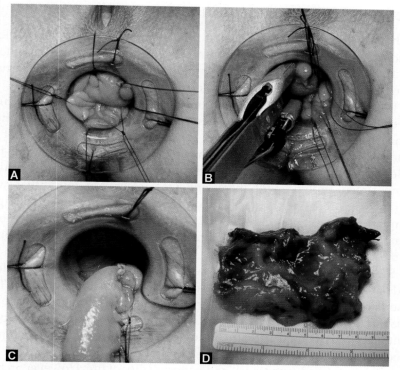

Figs 9.4A to D: (A) Transtar: a series of circumferential traction sutures are placed around the apex of the prolapse. (B) Full-thickness circumferential resection of the prolapse is performed with sequential firings of the Contour30 stapler. (C) The prolapse emerges from the CAD as a "sausage-shaped" specimen as the resection progresses. The opened specimen showing full-thickness resection of the distal rectum and mesorectal fat

rectal suspension (EXPRESS) procedure have been extended to internal rectal prolapse. A perineal dissection of the rectovaginal septum is performed and collagen mesh is attached to the anterolateral rectal walls, guided retropubically, and anchorage to the suprapubic periosteum, re-suspending the distal rectum. Although an interesting concept, the presently reported numbers are small with issues relating to frequent septic mesh complications.

Key Points

- Appropriate investigation and patient selection is paramount to successful outcomes when undertaking surgery for internal rectal prolapse.
- Two methods are described for STARR; PPH-STARR and Transtar. Current evidence does not favour one technique over the other.
- Combined pelvic organ prolapse surgery can be performed safely with benefits for healthcare providers and patients.

RECTAL AND OTHER PELVIC ORGAN PROLAPSE

Although it is not the intention of this chapter to present a complete description of pelvic organ prolapse, it would be incomplete to ignore the frequent association that rectal prolapse (full-thickness and internal) carries with other pelvic organ prolapse.

With an increasing emphasis on multidisciplinary working and specialised pelvic floor services, there is a trend to combined operating between coloproctologists and other pelvic floor surgeons. Babalola et al. found an increasing trend to multi-compartment repair particularly in the elderly,[37] which may be due to the increasing frequency of multi-compartment prolapse with increasing age. Hetzer et al. found that two-thirds of patients with faecal incontinence have evidence of triple compartment prolapse on radiological imaging and that surgery on one compartment alone leads to an increased risk of symptomatic prolapse in the remaining compartments.[38]

STARR can readily be combined with transvaginal repair to the middle and anterior compartments with the patient in the lithotomy position. The results of combined transanal and transvaginal procedures appear to be reasonable. Boccasanta et al. report results after two years follow-up of combined STARR and urogynaecological procedures.[39] The combined procedures were safe with effective restoration of normal anatomy on imaging, improved symptoms, and better quality of life. However, in this series STARR combined with hysterectomy was associated with a higher risk for complications and a longer inpatient stay than STARR alone or in combination with transobturator tape or transvaginal repair of an enterocele. The recurrence rates for urinary incontinence and vaginal vault prolapse were acceptable.

It is also possible to combine transabdominal procedures, such as laparoscopic sacrocolporectopexy, with other compartment repair either with the use of "Y" meshes or a separate transvaginal approach. The literature on combined transabdominal multi-compartment repair is sparse, involving small personal series with limited functional data and restricted to short-term outcome reporting. A combination of ventral rectopexy and colpohysteropexy in eight young patients has reported an improvement in overall symptoms in 87 per cent of cases, although the results in terms of improvement in constipation, either with or without sigmoid resection, were inconclusive.[40] A larger series of 18 patients undergoing laparoscopic ventral resectional rectopexy together with mesh vaginal vault sacropexy reported reasonable morbidity, but without functional outcomes.[41] The largest series of 23 patients undergoing rectal prolapse surgery in combination with urological or urogynaecological procedures showed it to be safe with similar outcome measures in terms of constipation and incontinence scores, quality of life and recurrence rates, as compared to rectal prolapse surgery alone.[42]

Thus, there is emerging evidence to support combined pelvic organ prolapse surgery. The argument for combined operating is really one of logistics, with benefits for both the healthcare provider and the patient derived from fewer hospital admissions, fewer general anaesthetics, less time off work, etc. The counter-argument in favour of a two-staged approach is that repair of one pelvic organ prolapse often has a secondary effect on the remaining two compartments, either for better or worse. If for the better, this may negate the need for a second intervention, whereas a detrimental effect may result to a change in operative procedure. There is a now a growing need for proper clinical trials to better understand the complex inter-relationships of pelvic organ prolapse and to rationalise our current approach.

Key Points for Clinical Practice

- In full-thickness rectal prolapse the doctrine of abdominal procedures for the medically fit and perineal procedures for the elderly and frail has been challenged by the introduction of laparoscopic techniques.
- In full-thickness rectal prolapse, laparoscopic ventral rectopexy offers benefits over posterior rectopexy in terms of better rectal autonomic nerve preservation and reduced postoperative constipation.
- Obstructed defaecation is the normal desire to defecate but an inability to satisfactorily evacuate the rectum. It is common in multiparous women.
- Both laparoscopic ventral rectopexy and STARR appear to be safe and effective in the treatment of obstructed defaecation associated with internal rectal prolapse.
- Appropriate investigation and patient selection is paramount to successful outcomes when undertaking surgery for internal rectal prolapse.
- Two methods are described for STARR; PPH-STARR and transtar. Current evidence does not favour one technique over the other. Combined pelvic organ prolapse surgery can be performed safely with benefits for healthcare providers and patients.

REFERENCES

1. Kupfer CA, Goligher JC. One hundred consecutive cases of complete rectal prolapse of the rectum treated by operation. Br J Surg 1970;57(7):482-7.
2. Nicholls JR, Banarjee A. Rectal prolapse and solitary rectal ulcer syndrome. In: Nicholls RJ, Dozois RR (Eds). Surgery of the Colon and Rectum. New York: Churchill Livingstone, 1997;709-37.
3. Senagore AJ. Management of rectal prolapse: The role of laparoscopic approaches. Seminars in Laparosc Surg 2003;10(4):197-202.
4. Tou S, Brown SR, Malik AI, et al. Surgery for complete rectal prolapse in adults. Cochrane Database of Systematic Reviews 2008;CD001758.
5. Speakman CTM, Madden MV, Nicholls RJ, et al. Lateral ligament division during rectopexy causes constipation but prevents recurrence: results of a prospective randomised study. Br J Surg 1991;78(12):1431-3.

6. Kellokumpu IH, Virozen J, Scheinin T. Laparoscopic repair of rectal prolapse: a prospective study evaluating surgical outcome and changes in symptoms and bowel function. Surg Endosc 2000;14(7):634-40.

7. Bruch HP, Herold A, Scheideck T, et al. Laparoscopic surgery for rectal prolapse and outlet obstruction. Dis Colon Rectum 1999;42(9):1189-94.

8. Blatchford GJ. Rectal prolapse: rational therapy without foreign material. Neth J Surg 1989;41(6):126-8.

9. Heah SM, Hartley J, Hurley J, et al. Laparoscopic suture rectopexy without resection is effective treatment for full-thickness rectal prolapse. Dis Colon Rectum 2000;43(5):638-43.

10. Benoist HP, Taffinder N, Gould S, et al. Functional results two years after laparoscopic rectopexy. Am J Surg 2001;182(2):168-73.

11. Samaranayake CB, Luo C, Plank AW, et al. Systematic review on ventral rectopexy for rectal prolapse and intussusception. Colorectal Dis 2010;12(6):504-12.

12. D'Hoore A, Cadoni R, Penninckx F. Long-term outcome of laparoscopic ventral rectopexy for total rectal prolapse. Br J Surg 2004;91(11):1500-5.

13. Tobin SA, Scott IHK. Delorme operation for rectal prolapse. Br J Surg 1994;81(11):1681-4.

14. Oliver GC, Vachon D, Eisenstat TE, et al. Delorme's procedure for complete rectal prolapse in severely debilitated patients: an analysis of 41 patients. Dis Colon Rectum 1994;37(5):461-7.

15. Watts AMI, Thompson MR. Evaluation of Delorme's procedure as a treatment for full-thickness rectal prolapse. Br J Surg 2000;87(2):218-22.

16. Yakut M, Kaymakciioglu N, Simsek A, et al. Surgical treatment of rectal prolapse: a retrospective analysis of 94 cases. Int Surg 1998;83(1):55-65.

17. Altemeier WA, Culbertson WR, Schwengerdt C, et al. Nineteen years' experience with the one-stage perineal repair of rectal prolapse. Ann Surg 1971;173(6):993-1006.

18. Ramanujam PS, Vankatesh KS, Fietz MJ. Perineal excision of rectal procidentia in elderly high-risk patients: a ten-year experience. Dis Colon Rectum 1994;37(10):1027-30.

19. Kim D-S, Tsang CB, Wong WD, et al. Complete rectal prolapse: evolution of management and results. Dis Colon Rectum 1999;42(4):460-9.

20. Scherer R, Marti L, Hetzer FH. Perineal stapled prolapse resection: a new procedure for external rectal prolapse. Dis Colon Rectum 2008;51(11):1727-30.

21. Hetzer FH, Roushan AH, Wolf K, et al. Functional outcome after perineal stapled prolapse resection for external rectal prolapse. BMC Surgery. 2010;10:9.

22. Collinson R, Wijffels N, Cunningham C, et al. Laparoscopic ventral rectopexy for internal rectal prolapse: short-term functional results. Colorectal Dis 2010;12(2):97-104.

23. Berman IR, Harris MS, Rabeler MB. Delorme's transanal excision for internal rectal prolapse: patient selection, technique, and three-year follow-up. Dis Colon Rectum 1990;33(7):573-80.

24. Orrom WJ, Bartolo DCC, Miller R, et al. Rectopexy is an ineffective treatment for obstructed defaecation. Dis Colon Rectum 1991;34(1):41-6.

25. Sarles JC, Arnaud A, Selezneff I, et al. Endo-rectal repair of rectocele. Int J Colorectal Dis 1989;4(3):167-71.

26. Berman IR, Manning DH, Dudley-Wright K. Anatomic specificity in the diagnosis and treatment of internal rectal prolapse. Dis Colon Rectum 1985;28(11):816-26.

27. Ripstein CB. Treatment of massive rectal prolapse. Am J Surg 1952;83(1): 68-71.

28. Slawik S, Soulsby R, Carter H, et al. Laparoscopic ventral rectopexy, posterior colporrhaphy and vaginal sacrocolpopexy for the treatment of recto-genital prolapse and mechanical outlet obstruction. Colorectal Dis 2008;10(2): 138-43.

29. D'Hoore A, Vanbeckevoort D, Penninckx F. Clinical, physical and radiological assessment of rectovaginal septum reinforcement with mesh for complex rectocele. Br J Surg 2008;95(10):1264-72.

30. Longo A. Treatment of hemorrhoidal disease by reduction of mucosa and hemorrhoidal prolapse with a circular suturing device: a new procedure. In: Proceedings of the 6th World Congress of Endoscopic Surgery. Bologna, Italy: Monduzzi Editore; 1998. pp. 777-84.

31. Wadhawan H, Shorthouse AJ, Brown SR. Surgery for obstructed defaecation: does the use of the Contour device (Trans-STARR) improve results? Colorectal Dis 2010;12(9):885-90.

32. Boccasanta P, Venturi M, Roviaro G. Stapled transanal rectal resection versus stapled anopexy in the cure of hemorrhoids associated with rectal prolapse. A randomized controlled trial. Int J Colorectal Dis. 2007;22(3):245-51.

33. Renzi A, Talento P, Giardiello C, et al. Stapled trans-anal rectal resection (STARR) by a new dedicated device for the surgical treatment of obstructed defaecation syndrome caused by rectal intussusception and rectocele: early results of a multicenter prospective study. Int J Colorectal Dis 2008;23(10): 999-1005.

34. Jayne DG, Schwandner O, Stuto A. Stapled transanal rectal resection for obstructed defaecation syndrome: one-year results of the European STARR Registry. Dis Colon Rectum. 2009;52(7):1205-12.

35. Schwandner O, Stuto A, Jayne D, et al. Decision-making algorithm for the STARR procedure in obstructed defecation syndrome: position statement of the group of STARR Pioneers. Surg Innov 2008;15(2):105-9.

36. Williams NS, Giordano P, Dvorkin LS, et al. External pelvic rectal suspension (the Express procedure) for full-thickness rectal prolapse: evolution of a new technique. Dis Colon Rectum 2005;48(2):307-16.

37. Babalola EO, Bharucha AE, Joseph Melton LJ 3rd, et al. Utilization of surgical procedures for pelvic organ prolapse: a population-based study in Olmsted County, Minnesota, 1965-2002. Int Urogynecol J Pelvic Floor Dysfunct 2008;19(19):1243–50.

38. Hetzer FH, Andreisek A, Tsagari C, et al. MR defecography in patients with fecal incontinence: imaging findings and their effect on surgical management. Radiology 2006;240(2):449-57.

39. Boccasanta P, Venturi M, Spennacchio M, et al. Prospective clinical and functional results of combined rectal and urogynecologic surgery in complex pelvic floor disorders. Am J Surg 2010;199(2):144-53.

40. Ayav A, Bresler L, Brunaud L,et al. Surgical management of combined rectal and genital prolapse in young patients: transabdominal approach. Int J Colorectal Dis 2005;20(2):173-9.

41. Grebe M, Thiel B, Bley K, et al. Vaginal prolapse and rectal obstruction. Treated with a vaginal vault mesh colpo suspension and laparoscopic resection rectopexy Chirurg. 2008;79(11):1072-6.

42. Riansuwan W, Hull TL, Bast J, et al. Combined surgery in pelvic organ prolapse is safe and effective. Colorectal Dis 2010;12(3):188-92.

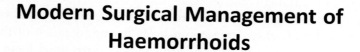

CHAPTER TEN

Modern Surgical Management of Haemorrhoids

Jonathan A McCullough, Deepak Singh-Ranger, Richard Cohen

INTRODUCTION

Haemorrhoids develop from naturally occurring anal cushions within the lower rectum. Commonly, there are three of these cushions are classically described as occupying the 3, 7 and 11 O'clock positions with the subject in the lithotomy position.[1] They are derived embryonically from rectal mucosal and submucosal folds, and derive their blood supply from the haemorrhoidal arteries, branches of the superior rectal arteries.

The three taeniae of the large bowel broaden over the sigmoid colon and invest the rectum in an outer layer of longitudinal muscle. This longitudinal muscle gives anchoring muscular extensions to the internal anal sphincter and to the anal cushions (Treitz's muscle) by keeping them in position and allowing them to function normally.[2]

Normal function of the anal cushions includes a 'washer' effect that allows complete closure of the rectal lumen, which could not be achieved by the muscular tube alone. The anal cushions are also involved in the rectoanal inhibitory reflex. Small amounts of rectal distension cause contraction of the external anal sphincter followed by relaxation of the internal anal sphincter. Described as a sampling mechanism by Jorge and Wexner[3] this reflex allows the anorectal junction to distinguish between solid, liquid and gas, and adjust continence accordingly. Indeed, the anal cushions contribute 15 to 20 per cent of anal resting pressure.[4]

PATHOPHYSIOLOGY

The muscular fibres of the anal canal and anal sphincters lie within a connective tissue matrix. Studies on juvenile cadavers and adult specimens[5] show that this matrix has a similar distribution in newborns and adults but the ratio of connective tissue: muscle changes with age, showing an increase in the amount of connective tissue. This leads to a loss in elasticity, allowing the anchoring muscle fibres that give support to the anal cushions and sphincter complex to fragment resulting in potential prolapse of haemorrhoidal tissue. Therefore, the development of haemorrhoids from the anal cushions may be seen as a natural progression of the aging process.

The common conception is that constipation and straining causes haemorrhoids although diarrhoea has also been shown to be a risk factor.[6] Certainly, spending long-periods of time sitting on the toilet with an unsupported and relaxed perineum leads to engorgement of the anal cushions and increases the downward shearing force upon them but in fact it should be pulled upwards during defaecation.[7] Coupled with the loss of supporting muscular fibres the venous plexus distends causing the haemorrhoids to bulge and descent follows.[8]

Haemorrhoids are common in the later stages of pregnancy and may be due to the gravid uterus causing compression on the pelvic venous system. Other risk factors including prolonged labour, long periods of straining, assisted deliveries, late delivery and large birth weight. As haemorrhoids usually regress in the post-partum period, 24 per cent in the first 3 months to 16 per cent after 6 months,[9] treatment should be aimed at prevention and symptom relief.

The vascular connections that form the porto-systemic shunt have been suggested as a possible mechanism for producing or enlarging haemorrhoids via portal obstruction and hypertension; however, the presenting pattern of troublesome haemorrhoids in patients with portal hypertension is no different to that of the general population. These patients have in fact a higher incidence of anorectal varices but these are a different anatomical entity.

PRESENTATION AND DIAGNOSIS

Haemorrhoids affect men and women equally but men are more likely to seek clinical treatment.[10] They are one of the most common anorectal conditions and one of the most common referrals to the general surgical clinic but their actual prevalence is largely unknown. Studies to ascertain their prevalence have suggested anywhere between 4.4 to 80 per cent of the population.[6,11,12] This wide range exists due to the large number of patients who may have haemorrhoids but are asymptomatic.

Haemorrhoids are most commonly classified by the traditional Goligher's grading of I to IV (Table 10.1). Skin tags may be present as a result of fibrosed external haemorrhoids or from stretch of the perianal skin. This classification only takes into account haemorrhoidal appearance rather than symptoms. Further attempts at classification include presenting symptoms and divide haemorrhoids into those that prolapse below the dentate line, termed external and those that swell, but remain above the dentate line, internal. A further distinction must also be made between circumferential haemorrhoids and the presence of skin tag remnants as this affects the choice of treatment.

TABLE 10.1

Goligher's classification of haemorrhoids

Grade I	Enlarged haemorrhoidal cushions
Grade II	Prolapse during defaecation and spontaneously reduce
Grade III	Prolapse during defaecation and must be manually reduced
Grade IV	Permanently prolapsed (thrombosed)

Additions of these extra classifications are unwieldy and therefore not commonly used. The surgeon must decide optimal treatment on a combination of appearance, anatomical position and symptoms.

Treatment should only be undertaken once all other causes of symptoms have been ruled out (e.g. IBD, rectal cancer) and if the patient is symptomatic.

Symptoms commonly described include bleeding, irritation, fullness, prolapse, difficult hygiene and seepage. These symptoms usually, but not always, depend upon the grade of haemorrhoid (Fig. 10.1). Likewise the severity of symptoms does not always correlate with the grade of haemorrhoid.

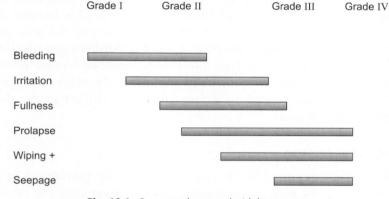

Fig. 10.1: Common haemorrhoidal symptoms

TREATMENT

Treatment depends upon the presenting symptoms and may be conservative, out-patient procedures or surgical operations under general or spinal anaesthesia.

Conservative Methods

Over the Counter Preparations

Mild haemorrhoidal symptoms are commonly treated by the General Practitioner or by self-medication. For many patients the first port of call is over the counter preparations such as soothing ointments containing mild astringents +/- local anaesthetic or compound ointments containing corticosteroids and local anaesthetic. While short-term results suggest an improvement in pain (90%), reduction in bleeding (50%) and relief of pruritus ani (80%); long-term data is lacking. These treatments give temporary relief and have been often tried before referral to the surgical clinic.

Out-Patient Clinic

Submucosal Sclerosant Injection

The most commonly used sclerosant is 5 per cent phenol in almond oil. Other sclerosants have been tried but their efficacy is not well-established. The sclerosant is injected into the submucosa just above the base of the haemorrhoid causing an inflammatory reaction and scarring just above the haemorrhoid. This is effective for haemorrhoids that bleed but not so for prolapsing haemorrhoids. There is no evidence to suggest that the repeated injections are beneficial. This is an easy method to perform in the OPD clinic and easy to teach; however, complications can occur, if the injection is too deep and prostatitis, urinary retention, and retroperitoneal sepsis have all been reported. For this reason, it is important to explain to the patient about the nature of the procedure and obtain at least verbal consent in case of out-patient setting. There is evidence that bulk laxatives alone may improve haemorrhoidal symptoms of bleeding and prolapse[13] and many clinicians now, prefer to give dietary and defecatory advice to patients suffering from early haemorrhoidal disease.

Rubber Band Ligation

Rubber band ligation (RBL) is popular and easily performed in the surgical clinic. The mechanism is similar to sclerosant injection, mucosa at the haemorrhoidal pedicle is grasped using a forceps passed through the banding device or using suction and a rubber band is deployed around the base of the grasped tissue (Fig. 10.2). This causes necrosis

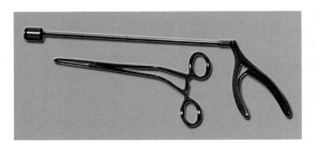

Fig.10.2: Haemorrhoidal banding

and scarring of the mucosa at the cranial aspect of the haemorrhoid which interrupts haemorrhoidal blood flow and tethers the haemorrhoid back into its functioning position.

This method has been shown to be the most successful non-surgical treatment[14] for haemorrhoids. It is particularly effective for Grade II haemorrhoids, but less so for Grade III with recurrence of symptoms being an issue.[15,16] One prospective study treating all grades of haemorrhoid with RBL showed 83 per cent of patients treated with bands were symptom-free at 2 months.[17] However, more than 50 per cent of patients complained of a recurrence of symptoms at one year follow-up. Comparison of RBL to excision haemorrhoidectomy (EH)[18] has shown no significant difference in the control of bleeding but there was more post-procedure associated pain with EH and no other difference between treatments in complication rate or patient satisfaction. EH showed a better overall cure rate with an 80 per cent less chance of symptom recurrence compared with RBL. EH success was higher for Grade III haemorrhoids with no significant superiority for Grade II.

The most common complications from banding are pain and haemorrhage occurring in up to 14 per cent of patients. Patients must be advised that there may be a post-procedural bleed for approximately 14 days which represents the sloughing off of the banded mucosa. Urinary retention, vaso-vagal episodes and life-threatening sepsis have also been reported.[19]

Key Points

- Haemorrhoids are one of the most common referrals to the surgical out-patient clinic symptoms do not always correlate with the size or grade of haemorrhoids
- Treatment should be tailored for each patient-based not only on the grade of haemorrhoid but also the symptoms and the degree of external tissue
- Other diseases such as bowel cancer and inflammatory bowel disease must be ruled out as a cause of symptoms before treatment is instigated.

Surgical Treatments

Haemorrhoidal Artery Ligation

Haemorrhoidal artery ligation is also known as Doppler guided haemorrhoidal artery ligation (DGHAL), transanal haemorrhoidal dearterialisation (THD) and haemorrhoidal artery ligation operation (HALO).

More recent techniques of treating haemorrhoids have sought to lessen the pain associated with excision haemorrhoidectomy, improve on recurrence rates associated with RBL and retain anatomical and physiological integrity of the anal cushions. First described in 1995.[20] DGHAL uses a modified proctoscope with a Doppler probe attachment (Fig. 10.3A and 3B) that identifies the position of haemorrhoidal arteries, allowing accurate ligation of the haemorrhoidal blood supply. This causes shrinkage and retraction of the anal cushion and if coupled with a plication stitch, treats the prolapsing element and returns the haemorrhoid to its original anatomical position. The advantage of this over EH is that

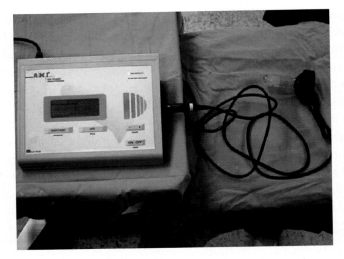

Fig. 10.3A: The haemorrhoid artery ligation operation equipment

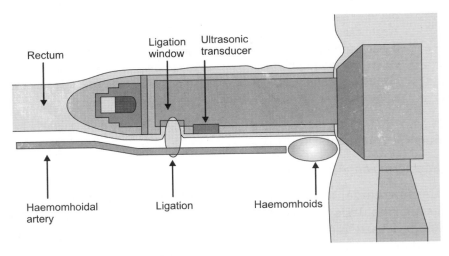

Fig.10.3B: Diagram showing artery ligation

surgery is performed in the insensate area above the dentate line, the haemorrhoid is not excised and therefore can contribute to continence.

Scheyer, et al.[21] reported a case series of 308 patients treated with DGHAL and classified their results according to the preoperative grade of haemorrhoid. At a median followup period of 18 months 6.7 per cent of patients with Grade II haemorrhoids, 13.5 per cent with Grade III haemorrhoids and 59.3 per cent of patients with Grade IV haemorrhoids had residual prolapse. Dal Monte, et al.[22] reported on 330 patients treated using this technique and also classified the results at one year based on the preoperative grade of haemorrhoid. They found a relapse rate of 4.8 per cent for Grade III haemorrhoids and 26.7 per cent for Grade IV haemorrhoids. In this study a patient subgroup was treated with either a plication or a figure-of-8 suture to the haemorrhoidal tissue, in addition to the arterial transfixion stitch. The recurrence rate for the plication stitch was 3.7 per cent for Grade III and 11.1 per cent for Grade IV haemorrhoids compared to 6 per cent for Grade III and 50 per cent for Grade IV in patients treated with a figure-of-8 stitch. Patient numbers in this subgroup study were small and the differences did not reach statistical significance. A recent prospective study has suggested this method be used on Grades I and II only.[23] Of 244 patients treated with DGHAL, 67 per cent had a satisfactory improvement of symptoms at follow-up. Of those receiving a second treatment of DGHAL or RBL only 46 per cent of the DGHAL patients reached a satisfactory improvement compared to 88 per cent of the RBL group. The study concluded that DGHAL be used for patients with Grade I or II haemorrhoids that are unresponsive to conservative methods. However, a systematic review of 17 studies by Giordano et al.[24] found a recurrence rate at one year is 10.8 per cent for prolapse, 9.7 per cent for bleeding and 8.7 per cent for pain at defecation. They concluded that this technique is useful for Grade II and III haemorrhoids.

Stapled Haemorrhoidopexy

Stapled haemorrhoidopexy is also known as Procedure for Prolapse and Haemorrhoids (PPH).

Stapling devices had previously been used in rectopexy procedures for prolapse and in rectal anastomoses. In 1998 Longo[25] first described the use of circular staplers for the treatment of prolapsing haemorrhoids. A circumferential suture is placed 2 cm above the haemorrhoidal tissue (Fig. 10.4 A). The anvil of the stapling gun (Ethicon Endo-Surgery, Inc.) is inserted and the suture pulled tight over the shaft of the gun (Fig. 10.4 B). The gun is then closed for 60 seconds and 'fired' which deploys an inner circular blade to excise a cylinder of mucosa and submucosa, and an outer series of staples to reconnect the mucosa. This system interrupts haemorrhoidal blood flow and retracts haemorrhoidal tissue to its original anatomical position (an anopexy). The procedure is designed to be less

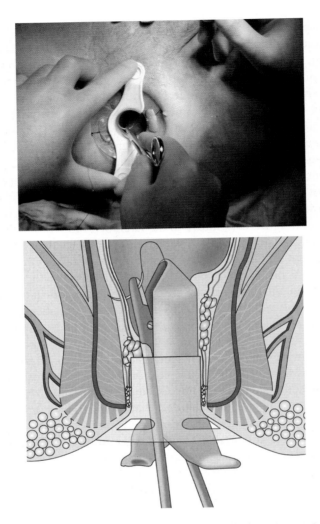

Fig.10.4A: Photograph and diagram of insertion of circumferential suture above haemorrhoids using the 'wingnut' proctoscope

painful than a surgical haemorrhoidectomy as the excised mucosa is from above the dentate line and the anal cushions are left intact.

Early studies showed that it had an advantage over EH for the treatment of Grade II and III haemorrhoids in terms of postoperative pain and time to return to work. It had a similar improvement in haemorrhoidal symptoms in the short-term.[26] Shalaby and Desoky[27] randomised 100 patients to EH or PPH and assessed symptoms at six months. Ninety-two per cent of patients treated with PPH were satisfied with their symptom improvement compared to 80 per cent in the surgical group. No proctological examination was performed at follow-up but pre

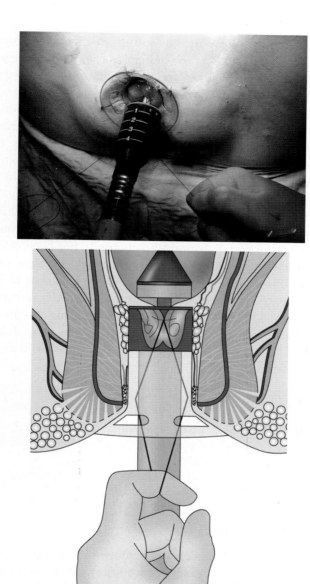

Fig.10.4B: Photograph and diagram showing the circumferential suture pulled tight over the shaft of the stapling gun (Ethicon Endo-Surgery)

and postoperative rectoanal manometry was performed in both groups of patients. This found a significant decrease in postoperative mean resting pressure and mean squeeze pressure in the surgical group, although no faecal incontinence was reported in either group.

149

However, longer follow-up has found an increased incidence of recurrence associated with PPH.[28] A randomised clinical trial comparing PPH with EH for Grade III and IV piles[29] found a significantly increased incidence of recurrence in the stapled group. Of interest, this recurrence was noted clinically from the fourth postoperative month onward. There was no significant difference in complications between the two methods. A meta-analysis of ten randomised controlled trials comparing these two procedures[30] found evidence in favour of PPH for operating time, hospital stay, postoperative pain and anal discharge. Skin tags and prolapse occurred at a higher rate following PPH and it was not found to be superior over EH in terms of postoperative bleeding, difficulty in defecating, anal fissure and stenosis, incontinence and sphincter damage.

Since its introduction, the surgical community has been divided over the use of PPH in treating haemorrhoids. A number of serious complications following PPH have been published including recto-vaginal fistulas, postoperative haemorrhage, perianal sepsis, retroperitoneal sepsis, colostomy formation and death. The reporting of complications following PPH may simply reflect awareness of a new procedure as these complications have been reported following other well-established treatments for haemorrhoids.[19]

Key Points

- All methods of treatment have potential complications. While these are rare, they are occasionally serious and must be discussed with the patient before any treatment is given
- Newer techniques have yet to establish themselves as more successful compared to more established procedures.

Surgical Haemorrhoidectomy

The practise of surgical excision of haemorrhoids has been present for centuries but the most popular technique for almost a century is the Milligan-Morgan 'excision-ligation' first described in 1937.[31] This classical technique uses scissors to excise the three anal cushions leaving a mucosal bridge between each wound to prevent anal stenosis. The cranial aspect of the cushion is ligated using an absorbable suture and the wounds are left open to heal by secondary intention (Fig. 10.5). The use of scissors has almost completely disappeared and the most popular subsequent modifications include diathermy and ligasure. In 1957 Ferguson[32] described the closed technique which was to improve postoperative pain and accelerate wound healing. There is some debate as to whether this technique is superior to the open form of haemorrhoidectomy[33,34] and it has not become common practise in the UK.

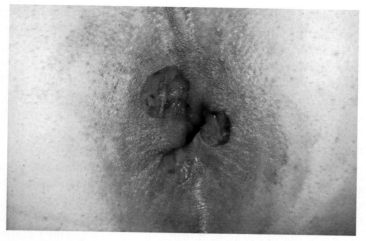

Fig.10.5: Postoperative 'Clover Leaf' following a Milligan-Morgan haemorrhoidectomy

There is no doubt that this procedure is painful and there has been concern regarding postoperative continence.[35] These potential complications have prompted the development of less painful and less invasive alternative procedures discussed above. However, due to the sustainability of results EH remains the gold standard treatment, particularly for Grades III and IV haemorrhoids.

Cochrane Collaborative Comparison of Treatments

In comparison to RBL, EH shown to be the superior treatment for Grade III haemorrhoids in long-term symptom control. This is at a price of greater postoperative pain, a higher complication rate and a longer-time to return to normal activity. There was little difference between the two treatments for Grade II haemorrhoids suggesting that RBL is the treatment of choice for Grade II and EH should be held in reserve for those whose symptoms recur following banding.[36]

The LigaSure ™ (Valleylab Inc., Boulder, Colorado, USA) system uses a high frequency current between its two blades that seals vessels. It has a minimal thermal spread of less than 2 mm which is thought to decrease the pain associated with EH. Early studies show comparable patient satisfaction compared with EH[37] and that it is as effective as a Milligan-Morgan procedure with a shorter operative time, decreased intra-operative blood loss,[38] reduced postoperative pain over the first two weeks[39] and a decrease in wound healing time.[40] Long-term data regarding recurrence of symptoms is lacking but the few studies published with longer-term follow-up show similar patient satisfaction, symptom control and incontinence scores.[41,42]

The stapled haemorrhoidopexy is described as an alternative to EH in the treatment of Grade III and IV piles. Long-term data[43] suggests that there is a greater recurrence of both haemorrhoids and symptoms, and an increased incidence of prolapse associated with the stapled technique. Although designed to be less painful and less invasive than EH the stapled technique does not show significant superiority in terms of pain, pruritus ani and faecal urgency. EH is considered as the gold standard treatment.

Our Own Practice

Grade I haemorrhoids treated conservatively with dietary and defecatory advice +/- the use of bulking laxatives, and in some cases injection sclerotherapy.

Grade II haemorrhoids are treated using the HALO device and we employ an absorbable plication suture with 2-0 vicryl as well as the vessel transfixion stitch. We also use this technique for Grade III haemorrhoids, but those with a large external component or bothersome external skin tags are treated with a Milligan-Morgan haemorrhoidectomy.

Grade IV haemorrhoids are treated with a Milligan-Morgan haemorrhoidectomy, if large skin tags are present, otherwise we use the PPH stapling technique. The stapled haemorrhoidopexy is also used for those patients with circumferential, prolapsing piles.

For Milligan-Morgan haemorrhoidectomies, we inject preoperatively 10 ml of 0.5 per cent marcaine intersphincterically and all patients are prescribed a 5 day course of metronidazole.[44] Patients undergoing excisional surgery are consented for either open or stapled haemorrhoidectomy, the decision being made at the time of examination under anaesthetic when a thorough assessment can be made.

NEW TECHNIQUES

The HemorPex System (HPS) is a single use device that resembles a proctoscope with a rotating, central axis that deploys a suture to ligate branches of the superior haemorrhoidal artery and a plication stitch to re-position the haemorrhoidal cushion. To date there is only one case series in the literature and comparison to established techniques is lacking.

Key Points for Clinical Practice

- Haemorrhoids are one of the most common referrals to the surgical out-patient clinic symptoms do not always correlate with the size or grade of haemorrhoids
- Treatment should be tailored for each patient-based not only on the grade of haemorrhoid but also the symptoms and the degree of external tissue
- Other diseases such as bowel cancer and inflammatory bowel disease must be ruled out as a cause of symptoms before treatment is instigated.

- All methods of treatment have potential complications. While these are rare, they are occasionally serious and must be discussed with the patient before any treatment is given
- Newer techniques have yet to establish themselves as more successful compared to more established procedures.

REFERENCES

1. Thomson WHF. The nature of haemorrhoids. Br J Surg 1975;62(7):542-52.
2. Lunniss PJ, Mann CV. Classification of internal haemorrhoids: a discussion paper. Colorectal Dis 2004;6(4):226-32.
3. Jorge JM, Wexner SD. Anorectal manometry: techniques and clinical applications. South Med J 1993;86(8):924-31.
4. Lestar B, Penninckx F, Kerremans R. The composition of anal basal pressure. An *in vivo* and *in vitro* study in man. Int J Colorectal Dis 1989;4(2):118-22.
5. Haas PA, Fox TA. Age-related changes and scar formations of perianal connective tissue. Dis Colon Rectum 1980;23(3):160-9.
6. Johansen JF, Sonnenberg A. Constipation is not a risk factor for haemorrhoids: a case-controlled study of potential etiological agents. Am J Gastroenterol 1994;89:1981-6.
7. Shafik A. A new concept of the anatomy of the anal sphincter mechanism and the physiology of defecation III. The longitudinal anal muscle: anatomy and role in sphincter mechanism. Invest Urol 1976;13(4):271-7.
8. Haas PA, Fox TA, Haas GP. The pathogenesis of haemorrhoids. Dis Colon Rectum 1984;27(7):442-50.
9. Avsar AF, Keskin HL. Haemorrhoids during pregnancy. J Obstet Gynaecol 2010;30(3):231-7.
10. Hussain JN. Haemorrhoids. Prim Care 1999;26(1):35-51.
11. Gazet JC, Redding W, Rickett JW. The prevalence of haemorrhoids. A preliminary survey. Proc R Soc Med 1970;63:78-80.
12. Haas PA, Haas GP, Schmaltz S, et al. The prevalence of haemorrhoids. Dis Colon Rectum 1983;26(7):435-9.
13. Senapati A, Nicholls RJ. A randomised trial to compare the results of injection sclerotherapy with a bulk laxative alone in the treatment of bleeding haemorrhoids. Int J Colorect Dis 1988;3(2):124-6.
14. MacRae HM, McLeod RS. Comparison of haemorrhoidal treatment modalities. A meta-analysis. Dis Colon Rectum 1995;38(7):687-94.
15. Murie JA, Mackenzie I, Sim AJ. Rubber band ligation versus haemorrhoidectomy for prolapsing haemorrhoids: a long-term prospective clinical trial. Br J Surg 1982;69(9):536-8.
16. Lewis AA, Rogers HS, Leighton M. Trial of maximal anal dilation, cryotherapy and elastic band ligation as alternatives to haemorrhoidectomy in the treatment of large prolapsing haemorrhoids. Br J Surg 1983;70(1):54-6.
17. Longman RJ, Thomson WH. A prospective study of outcome from rubber band ligation of piles. Colorectal Dis 2005;8(2):145-8.

18. Shanmugam V, Thaha MA, Rabindranath KS, et al. Systematic review of randomized trials comparing rubber band ligation with excisional haemorrhoidectomy. Br J Surg 2005;92(12):1481-7.

19. McCloud JM, Jameson JS, Scott AN. Life-threatening sepsis following treatment for haemorrhoids: a systematic review. Colorectal Dis 2006;8(9):748-55.

20. Morinaga K, Hasuda K, Ikeda T. A novel therapy for internal hemorrhoids: ligation of the hemorrhoidal artery with a newly devised instrument (Moricorn) in conjunction with a Doppler flowmeter. Am J Gastroenterol 1995;90(4):610-3.

21. Scheyer M, Antonietti E, Rollinger G, et al. Doppler-guided hemorrhoidal artery ligation. Am J Surg 2006;191(1):89-93.

22. Dal Monte PP, Tagariello C, Sarago M, et al. Transanal haemorrhoidal dearterialisation: nonexcisional surgery for the treatment of haemorrhoidal disease. Tech Coloproctol 2007;11(4):338-8.

23. Pol RA, van der Zwet WC, Hoornenborg D, et al. Results of 244 consecutive patients with hemorrhoids treated with Doppler-guided hemorrhoidal artery ligation. Dig Surg 2010;27(4):279-84.

24. Giordano P, Overton J, Madeddu F, et al. Transanal haemorrhoidal dearterialisation: a systematic review. Dis Colon Rectum 2009;52:1665-71.

25. Longo A. Treatment of haemorrhoidal disease by reduction of mucosa and haemorrhoidal prolapse with a circular suturing device: a new procedure. Proceedings of the 6th World Congress of Endoscopic Surgery. Rome 1998;777-84.

26. Mehigan BJ, Motson JRT, Hartley JE. Stapling procedure for haemorrhoids versus Milligan-Morgan haemorrhoidectomy: randomised controlled trial. Lancet 2000;355(9206):782-5.

27. Shalaby R, Desoky A. Randomized clinical trial of stapled versus Milligan-Morgan hemorrhoidectomy. Br J Surg 2001;88(8):1049-53.

28. Nisar PJ, Acheson AG, Neal KR, et al. Stapled haemorrhoidopexy compared with conventional haemorrhoidectomy: systematic review of randomised, controlled trials. Dis Colon Rectum 2004;47:1837-45.

29. Ortiz H, Marzo J, Armendariz P. Randomized clinical trial of stapled haemorrhoidopexy versus conventional diathermy haemorrhoidectomy. Br J Surg 2002;89(11):1376-81.

30. Lan P, Wu X, Zhou X, et al. The safety and efficacy of stapled hemorrhoidectomy in the treatment of hemorrhoids: a systematic review and meta-analysis of ten randomized control trials. Int J Colorectal Dis 2006;21(2):172-8.

31. Milligan ETC, Morgan CN, Officer R, et al. Surgical anatomy of the anal canal, and the operative treatment of haemorrhoids. Lancet 1937;ii:119-24.

32. Ferguson DJ, Heaton JR. Closed hemorrhoidectomy. Dis Colon Rectum 1959;2(2):176-9.

33. Ho YH, Seow-Choen F, Tan M, et al. Randomized controlled trial of open and closed haemorrhoidectomy. Br J Surg 1997;84(12):1729-30.

34. Arroyo A, Perez F, Miranda E, et al. Open versus closed day-case haemorrhoidectomy: is there any difference? Results of a prospective randomised study. Int J Colorectal Dis 2004;19(4):370-3.

35. Bennett RC, Friedman MH, Goligher JC. The late results of haemorrhoidectomy by ligature and excision. Br Med J 1962;2(5351):216-9.
36. Shanmugam V, Thaha MA, Rabindranath KS, et al. Rubber band ligation versus excisional haemorrhoidectomy for haemorrhoids. Cochrane Database Syst Rev 2005;(3):CD005034.
37. Palazzo FF, Francis DL, Clifton MA. Randomized clinical trial of Ligasure versus open haemorrhoidectomy. Br J Surg 2002;89(2):154-7.
38. Jayne DG, Botterill I, Ambrose NS, et al. Randomized clinical trial of Ligasure versus conventional diathermy for day-case haemorrhoidectomy. Br J Surg 2002;89(4):428-32.
39. Nienhujis SW, de Hingh I. Conventional versus LigaSure haemorrhoidectomy for patients with symptomatic haemorrhoids. Cochrane Database of Systematic Reviews 2009;(1):CD006761.
40. Milito G, Cadeddu F, Muzi MG, et al. Haemorrhoidectomy with Ligasure vs. conventional excisional techniques: meta-analysis of randomized controlled trials. Colorectal Dis 2010;12(2):85-93.
41. Lawes DA, Palazzo FF, Francis DL, et al. One year follow up of a randomized trial comparing Ligasure with open haemorrhoidectomy. Colorectal Dis 2004;6(4):233-5.
42. Peters CJ, Botterill I, Ambrose NS, et al. Ligasure vs conventional diathermy haemorrhoidectomy: long-term follow-up of a randomised clinical trial. Colorectal Dis 2005;7(4):350-3.
43. Lumb KJ, Colquhoun PHD, Malthaner R, et al. Stapled versus conventional surgery for haemorrhoids. Cochrane Database of Sys Rev 2006;(4):CD005393.
44. Carapeti EA, Kamm MA, McDonald PJ, et al. Double-blind randomised controlled trial of effect of metronidazole on pain after day-case haemorrhoidectomy. Lancet 1998;351(9097):169-72.

SECTION FOUR

BREAST

CHAPTER ELEVEN

Radiotherapy for the Breast Surgeon

Dibor C, Douek M

INTRODUCTION

Over the last three decades, there has been a shift away from radical surgery towards breast conserving surgery without a detrimental effect on overall survival, so long as patients receive adjuvant postoperative radiotherapy.[1,2] The ultimate goal of breast cancer treatment remains improving survival, but with significant improvements in therapy, increasing emphasis is now placed on reducing treatment related morbidity and improving quality of life. With the introduction of sentinel lymph node biopsy (SLNB), axillary surgery has also become more targeted and conservative in women with a clinically and radiologically normal axilla. This change significantly reduced the morbidity associated with axillary node dissection.[3]

There is now a growing interest in alternative methods of delivering adjuvant radiotherapy that can reduce the morbidity, but maintain the therapeutic benefit. Over the last decade attempts have been made to reduce the size of the radiation field, reduce the number of treatment fractions needed and evaluate different modes of delivering radiotherapy. The main advances in adjuvant radiotherapy include the introduction of several methods for partial breast irradiation (PBI), hypofractionated accelerated breast radiotherapy and clarification of the indications for post-mastectomy radiotherapy.

EXTERNAL BEAM RADIOTHERAPY

Whole Breast Radiotherapy

Adjuvant whole breast radiotherapy after breast conserving surgery has been shown to significantly reduce local recurrence following breast conserving surgery, and by doing so, to improve overall survival in the longer term.[4] Adjuvant endocrine treatment and chemotherapy also have a beneficial effect on the risk of local recurrence. For instance, in patients with oestrogen-receptor (ER) positive breast cancer, five years of adjuvant tamoxifen reduces the risk of local recurrence by about one half (local recurrence rate ratio 0.47) and with adjuvant chemotherapy, by about one-third, irrespective of ER status.[4] In patients with human epidermal growth factor receptor 2 (HER2) positive breast cancer, the risk of local recurrence is also dramatically reduced which may have implications on the optimal delivery of radiotherapy, in the future.

Conventionally, whole breast radiotherapy is given in fractionated doses, five days a week over a five week period (50 Gy over 25 fractions).[5] This is followed by a boost to the tumour bed over a further 1–2 weeks, for higher risk tumours (e.g. age <40 years, grade III, lymph node involvement). This is largely based on the EORTC 22881-10882 trial[6] which demonstrated that a boost of 16 Gy to the tumour bed improved local recurrence rate, but not survival. In patients with heavy axillary nodal involvement (>4 involved nodes), additional radiotherapy to the supraclavicular fossa is indicated. Routine radiotherapy to the axilla after axillary dissection should be avoided since it significantly increases morbidity. For ductal carcinoma in-situ (DCIS), there is evidence that postoperative whole breast radiotherapy following breast conserving surgery, improves disease-free survival, but there is no evidence that it improves overall survival.[7,8]

Adjuvant radiotherapy treatment usually commences after the surgical wound has healed (over four weeks) and a delay of over eight weeks from surgery, can increase the local recurrence rate at five years.[9] Since breast cancer is very common, adjuvant radiotherapy for breast cancer can amount to 30% of the workload of radiotherapy departments. This can cause a delay in the commencement of adjuvant radiotherapy due to prolonged treatment waiting times. In patients who require adjuvant chemotherapy, radiotherapy is deferred until after chemotherapy which also leads to a delay in the delivery of adjuvant radiotherapy.

Hypofractionated Radiotherapy Regimens

Following the introduction of breast conserving surgery, hypofractionated regimens were common since the number of patients requiring adjuvant radiotherapy rose rapidly and radiotherapy waiting times lengthened. It later became evident that hypofractionated regimens caused greater morbidity largely due to routine coverage of the axilla and supraclavicular fossa.[10] Adjuvant radiotherapy to the breast only is now common practice and the equivalence of hypofractionated schedules compared to the traditional regimen (50 Gy in 25 fractions), has been demonstrated in randomised controlled trials.[11,12] The UK START trials A[13] and B[14] found that a radiotherapy schedule of 41.6 Gy in 13 fractions and 40 Gy in 15 fractions, respectively, offer rates of loco-regional tumour relapse and late adverse effects at least as favourable as the standard schedule of 50 Gy in 25 fractions. A further five fractions as a boost to the tumour bed, are usually administered following the results of the European Organization for Research and Treatment of Cancer (EORTC) boost trial.[15]

Post-mastectomy Radiotherapy

Post-mastectomy radiotherapy to the chest wall, reduces loco-regional recurrence and improves overall survival in high-risk (involvement of one or more lymph node, tumour size > 5 cm, skin or pectoral fascia involvement) pre-menopausal women with breast cancer.[16,17] Although post-mastectomy radiotherapy is offered to patients with four or more involved nodes, controversy still exists over the benefit of adjuvant radiotherapy post-mastectomy in patients with 1–3 involved nodes. The latter is addressed by the UK Medical Research Council (MRC), **S**elective **U**se of **P**ostoperative **R**adiotherapy aft**E**r **M**astect**O**my *(SUPREMO)* trial.

The likelihood of requiring postoperative radiotherapy can affect the choice of immediate breast reconstruction. Following immediate breast reconstruction, post-mastectomy radiotherapy planning is often compromised which may lead to reduced chest wall coverage, less effective coverage of the ipsilateral internal mammary chain and less effective lung minimization.[18] Immediate reconstruction and associated complications may also contribute to a delay in commencement of adjuvant radiotherapy, beyond the acceptable eight weeks after surgery.[9] With the increasing use of skin-sparing mastectomy, subcutaneous (nipple-sparing) mastectomy and acellular tissue dermal substitutes for breast implant reconstruction, the indications for immediate breast reconstruction prior to post-mastectomy radiotherapy, should be reconsidered. A literature review by Namrata et al.[19] suggests that delayed reconstruction has a superior cosmetic outcome and less late complications (e.g. fat necrosis, flap volume loss, contracture) compared to immediate reconstruction. This needs to be balanced against the psychological advantages of an immediate reconstruction and therefore, the optimal type of reconstruction needs to be tailored to the individual patient taking into consideration the likelihood of requiring subsequent adjuvant radiotherapy.

Intensity Modulated Radiotherapy (IMRT)

Intensity modulated radiotherapy is not widely used in breast cancer. Partial breast radiotherapy can be delivered using intensity modulated radiotherapy. This is currently the subject of clinical trials including the UK IMPORT and the National Surgical Adjuvant Breast and Bowel Project (NSABP) B39 trials (3D conformal).[20]

External beam radiotherapy relies on patients living within reach of a linear accelerator and can raise practical and or financial difficulties to patients who live a long distance away. In some countries, patients may decline radiotherapy and in others may even opt for mastectomy in an attempt to avoid radiotherapy. There is thus a clinical need for alternative radiotherapy treatment options that shorten the duration and intensity of treatment.

Partial Breast Radiotherapy

The application of local radiotherapy to the breast is not new. In 1937, Sir Geoffrey Keynes reported the use of radium needles to deliver local radiotherapy to the breast and this predates the introduction of super high voltage external beam radiotherapy. Over the last decade there has been a growing interest in local radiotherapy treatment to the operated cavity or index quadrant in addition to IMRT. This resulted from the observation that over 90% of local recurrences from breast cancer occur at the index (operated) quadrant,[21,22] and this is in stark contrast to the observation that cancer foci can frequently be seen away from the index quadrant in mastectomy specimens.[23,24] Thus, the need for whole breast radiotherapy and its associated morbidity, has been questioned. Several trials are now underway to assess the efficacy of PBI administered to the operated quadrant intra-operatively, or to the index quadrant in the immediate postoperative period. These techniques are used to deliver radiotherapy either directly to the tumour bed or to the index quadrant.

A recent meta-analysis of the existing trials of PBI [prior to publication of the targeted intraoperative radio-therapy (TARGIT) trial], concluded that PBI is associated with a small increase in local recurrence without a detrimental effect on overall survival.[25]

Intraoperative Radiotherapy

Intraoperative radiotherapy is delivered as a single fraction at the time of the cancer operation, or at a subsequent second procedure. The intrabeam system (Carl Zeiss, Oberkochen, Germany) is used to deliver a single fraction of radiotherapy during surgery (Figs 11.1A to B), to the tumour bed. The device delivers electron generated low energy X-rays (50 kV maximum) at the tip of a 3.2 mm diameter tube that is placed at the centre of a spherical applicator. Different sizes of spherical applicators (1.5–5 cm) are available and the optimal size is used to fit the operated cavity. A total of 20 Gy is delivered at the surface of the applicator over 20–35 minutes. Once the applicator is in place, sutures are used in a "purse string" formation to make the breast tissue conform to the surface and shape of the applicator. In the TARGIT-A trial, over 2,232 patients were randomised to either intra-operative radiotherapy (IORT) or external beam radiotherapy.[26] After four years median follow-up, there were six recurrences in the IORT and five in the external beam arms, demonstrating non-inferiority. Radiotherapy toxicity was significantly lower in the IORT arm.

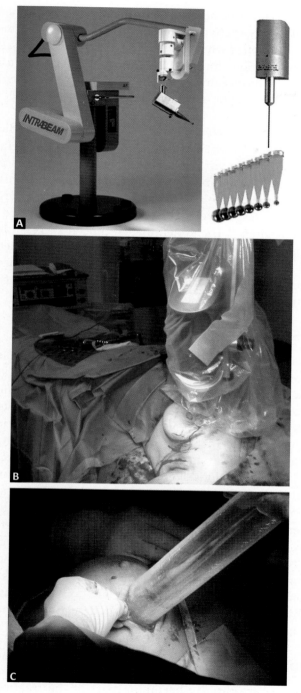

Figs 11.1A to C: (A) The Intrabeam system for delivering intraoperative radiotherapy has a gantry that facilitates positioning of the radiotherapy device. In the theatre (B) electron-generated radiotherapy is delivered via the optimal sized spherical applicator, inserted into the tumour bed. (C) In the ELIOT trial, a collimator is used to deliver radiotherapy intra-operatively.

163

Intraoperative radiotherapy could also replace the need for the conventional postoperative radiotherapy boost to the tumour bed,[27] reducing the duration of whole breast radiotherapy. Future trials will need to refine the indications for IORT as a form of PBI and as a boost. The advantages of the Intrabeam system includes, ease of use, single fraction, no need for lead-lining of operating theatres and low cost compared to external beam.

Another randomised controlled trial of intraoperative radiotherapy is the ELIOT trial, developed in Milan.[28] A mobile linear accelerator is used to deliver radiotherapy via a collimator (Fig. 11.1C). In a large series of off-trial patients,[29] the feasibility of this technique was demonstrated with a low local recurrence rate of 2.3% and 5 and 10 years survival rates of 97.4% and 89.7%, respectively. The results of the randomised controlled trial are still awaited.[30] The system has also been successfully used for on-table nipple-areolar complex irradiation during subcutaneous (nipple sparing) mastectomy.[31] Disadvantages of ELIOT include the need for lead-lining of operating theatres, need for pectoral fascial dissection, chest-wall shielding and higher equipment costs.

Brachytherapy

Brachytherapy is a form of radiotherapy in which the radiation source is placed inside the breast. A randomised controlled trial (n = 258) of a high dose rate (HDR) multicatheter brachytherapy device, showed a higher actuarial five years local recurrence rate (4.7% vs 3.4%) but no difference in overall survival.[32] The commonest device in use is the MammoSite (Hologic Inc, Bedford, USA) which is composed of a balloon catheter that is left in the tumour bed. Subsequent radiotherapy is delivered as five fractions over five days. Since breast drains are now infrequently used, the requirement of an indwelling catheter is a drawback of this technique. Furthermore, a 7 mm minimum distance is recommended from the skin surface to the balloon catheter, to avoid irradiating the overlying skin. Lead-lined operating theatres or treatment rooms must be used for safe practice. Since the Food and Drug Administration (FDA) approval of this device, there is an ongoing non-randomised prospective registry trial[33] to gather outcome data. The NSABP B39[20] randomised controlled trial, also includes this technique amongst a number of different techniques of PBI.

CONCLUSION

PBI techniques are rapidly becoming part of the treatment options available for adjuvant radiotherapy. The combination of breast conserving surgery, sentinel node biopsy and PBI further reduce morbidity associated with breast cancer surgery. IMRT is still not widely accepted for breast cancer adjuvant radiotherapy, but ongoing studies may demonstrate that it is useful in treating node-positive breast cancer when wide-field nodal targets need to be included in the treatment volume. Future trials of PBI will need to evaluate more specific indications for PBI, the optimal delivery schedule and optimum dose. Partial breast IMRT and image-guided radiotherapy (IGRT) may prove to be acceptable techniques for PBI, although reliance on more imaging for treatment planning and longer treatment schedule compared to other types of PBI, may prove to be a significant drawback.

Key Points for Clinical Practice

- Adjuvant whole breast radiotherapy after breast conserving surgery has been shown to significantly reduce local recurrence following breast conserving surgery, and by doing so, to improve overall survival in the longer term.
- There is now a growing interest in alternative methods of delivering adjuvant radiotherapy for breast cancer that can reduce the morbidity but maintain the therapeutic benefit.
- The main advances in adjuvant radiotherapy include the introduction of several methods for partial breast irradiation (PBI), hypofractionated accelerated breast radiotherapy and clarification of the indications for post-mastectomy radiotherapy.
- Adjuvant radiotherapy treatment usually commences after the surgical wound has healed (over 4 weeks) and a delay of over 8 weeks from surgery, can increase the local recurrence rate at 5 years.
- The TARGIT-A trial demonstrated that for selected patients with early breast cancer, intraoperative radiotherapy should be considered as an alternative to external beam radiotherapy. A recent meta-analysis of the existing trials of PBI, prior to publication of the TARGIT trial, concluded that PBI is associated with a small increase in local recurrence without a detrimental effect on overall survival.

REFERENCES

1. Fisher B, Anderson S, Bryant J, et al. Twenty-year follow-up of a randomized trial comparing total mastectomy, lumpectomy, and lumpectomy plus irradiation for the treatment of invasive breast cancer. N Engl J Med 2002;347(16):1233-41.
2. Veronesi U, Cascinelli N, Mariani L, et al. Twenty-year follow-up of a randomized study comparing breast-conserving surgery with radical mastectomy for early breast cancer. N Engl J Med 2002;347(16):1227-32.
3. Mansel RE, Fallowfield L, Kissin M, et al. Randomized multicenter trial of sentinel node biopsy versus standard axillary treatment in operable breast cancer: the ALMANAC Trial. J Natl Cancer Inst 2006;98(9):599-609.
4. Clarke M, Collins R, Darby S, et al. Effects of radiotherapy and of differences in the extent of surgery for early breast cancer on local recurrence and 15-year survival: an overview of the randomised trials. Lancet 2005; 366(9503):2087-106.

5. CG80 Early and locally advanced breast cancer: full guidance; 2009.

6. Bartelink H, Horiot JC, Poortmans PM, et al. Impact of a higher radiation dose on local control and survival in breast-conserving therapy of early breast cancer: 10-year results of the randomized boost versus no boost EORTC 22881-10882 trial. J Clin Oncol 2007;25(22):3259-65.

7. Fisher B, Dignam J, Wolmark N, et al. Lumpectomy and radiation therapy for the treatment of intraductal breast cancer: findings from National Surgical Adjuvant Breast and Bowel Project B-17. J Clin Oncol 1998;16(2): 441-52.

8. Bijker N, Meijnen P, Peterse JL, et al. Breast-conserving treatment with or without radiotherapy in ductal carcinoma-in-situ: ten-year results of European Organisation for Research and Treatment of Cancer randomized phase III trial 10853—a study by the EORTC Breast Cancer Cooperative Group and EORTC Radiotherapy Group. J Clin Oncol 2006;24(21):3381-7.

9. Huang J, Barbera L, Brouwers M, et al. Does delay in starting treatment affect the outcomes of radiotherapy? A systematic review. J Clin Oncol 2003;21(3):555-63.

10. Powell S, Cooke J, Parsons C. Radiation-induced brachial plexus injury: follow-up of two different fractionation schedules. Radiother Oncol 1990;18(3):213-20.

11. Haviland JS, Yarnold JR, Bentzen SM. Hypofractionated radiotherapy for breast cancer. N Engl J Med 2010;362(19):1843-4.

12. Whelan TJ, Pignol JP, Levine MN, et al. Long-term results of hypo-fractionated radiation therapy for breast cancer. N Engl J Med 2010;362(6): 513-20.

13. Bentzen SM, Agrawal RK, Aird EG, et al. The UK Standardisation of Breast Radiotherapy (START) Trial A of radiotherapy hypofractionation for treatment of early breast cancer: a randomised trial. Lancet Oncol 2008;9(4):331-41.

14. Bentzen SM, Agrawal RK, Aird EG, et al. The UK Standardisation of Breast Radiotherapy (START) Trial B of radiotherapy hypofractionation for treatment of early breast cancer: a randomised trial. Lancet 2008;371(9618): 1098-107.

15. Bartelink H, Horiot JC, Poortmans P, et al. Recurrence rates after treatment of breast cancer with standard radiotherapy with or without additional radiation. N Engl J Med 2001;345(19):1378-87.

16. Overgaard M, Hansen PS, Overgaard J, et al. Postoperative radiotherapy in high-risk premenopausal women with breast cancer who receive adjuvant chemotherapy. Danish Breast Cancer Cooperative Group 82b Trial. N Engl J Med 1997;337(14):949-55.

17. Ragaz J, Jackson SM, Le N, et al. Adjuvant radiotherapy and chemotherapy in node-positive premenopausal women with breast cancer. N Engl J Med 1997;337(14):956-62.

18. Motwani SB, Strom EA, Schechter NR, et al. The impact of immediate breast reconstruction on the technical delivery of postmastectomy radiotherapy. Int J Radiat Oncol Biol Phys 2006;66(1):76-82.

19. Anavekar NS, Rozen WM, Le Roux CM, et al. Achieving autologous breast reconstruction for breast cancer patients in the setting of post-mastectomy radiotherapy. J Cancer Surviv 2010.

20. Bovi J, Qi XS, White J, et al. Comparison of three accelerated partial breast irradiation techniques: treatment effectiveness based upon biological models. Radiother Oncol 2007;84(3):226-32.

21. Veronesi U, Luini A, Del Vecchio M, et al. Radiotherapy after breast-preserving surgery in women with localized cancer of the breast. N Engl J Med 1993;328(22):1587-91.

22. Fisher ER, Anderson S, Redmond C, et al. Ipsilateral breast tumor recurrence and survival following lumpectomy and irradiation: pathological findings from NSABP protocol B-06. Semin Surg Oncol 1992;8(3):161-6.

23. Baum M, Vaidya JS, Mittra I. Multicentricity and recurrence of breast cancer. Lancet 1997;349(9046):208.

24. Douek M, Vaidya JS, Lakhani SR, et al. Can magnetic-resonance imaging help elucidate natural history of breast cancer multicentricity? Lancet 1998;351(9105):801-2.

25. Valachis A, Mauri D, Polyzos NP, et al. Partial breast irradiation or whole breast radiotherapy for early breast cancer: a meta-analysis of randomized controlled trials. Breast J 2010;16(3):245-51.

26. Vaidya JS, Joseph DJ, Tobias JS, et al. Targeted intraoperative radiotherapy versus whole breast radiotherapy for breast cancer (TARGIT-A trial): an international, prospective, randomised, non-inferiority phase 3 trial. Lancet 2010;376(9735):91-102.

27. Vaidya JS, Baum M, Tobias JS, et al. Targeted intraoperative radiotherapy (TARGIT) yields very low recurrence rates when given as a boost. Int J Radiat Oncol Biol Phys 2006;66(5):1335-8.

28. Orecchia R, Ciocca M, Lazzari R, et al. Intraoperative radiation therapy with electrons (ELIOT) in early-stage breast cancer. Breast 2003;12(6):483-90.

29. Veronesi U, Orecchia R, Luini A, et al. Intraoperative radiotherapy during breast conserving surgery: a study on 1,822 cases treated with electrons. Breast Cancer Res Treat 2010;124(1):141-51.

30. Intra M, Luini A, Gatti G, et al. Surgical technique of intraoperative radiation therapy with electrons (ELIOT) in breast cancer: a lesson learned by over 1000 procedures. Surgery 2006;140(3):467-71.

31. Petit JY, Veronesi U, Orecchia R, et al. Nipple-sparing mastectomy in association with intra operative radiotherapy (ELIOT): A new type of mastectomy for breast cancer treatment. Breast Cancer Res Treat 2006;96(1): 47-51.

32. Polgar C, Fodor J, Major T, et al. Breast-conserving treatment with partial or whole breast irradiation for low-risk invasive breast carcinoma—5-year results of a randomized trial. Int J Radiat Oncol Biol Phys 2007;69(3):694-702.

33. Beitsch P, Vicini F, Keisch M, et al. Five-year outcome of patients classified in the "unsuitable" category using the American Society of Therapeutic Radiology and Oncology (ASTRO) Consensus Panel guidelines for the application of accelerated partial breast irradiation: an analysis of patients treated on the American Society of Breast Surgeons MammoSite(R) Registry trial. Ann Surg Oncol 2010;17(Suppl 3):219-25.

CHAPTER TWELVE

An Update on the Management of the Axilla in Breast Cancer

Hill ADK, McHugh SM, Corrigan MA

INTRODUCTION

Controversy persists regarding the optimal management of the axilla in breast cancer. The accurate assessment of axillary lymph nodes (ALNs) provides staging information essential to the optimal treatment of breast cancer patients.

This chapter reviews current management of the axilla in breast cancer taking into account recent changes which have evolved in clinical practice from both a diagnostic and therapeutic perspective.

DIAGNOSING DISEASE OF THE AXILLA

Accurate assessment of axillary nodal status remains the most important prognostic factor for patients with breast cancer.[1] Mapping of ALNs and sentinel lymph nodes (SLNs) biopsy is widely-used, clinically preferred and minimally invasive procedure for the identification of lymph node metastasis.[2] The SNL is defined as the first draining lymph node on the direct lymphatic pathway from the primary tumour site[3] and as such is the first node to harbour cancer cells detached from the primary tumour. An intricate system of lymphatic channels draining the breast usually converge towards a group of three to five nodes in the axilla, classified as SLNs.

Key Point

- Axillary node involvement is the most important prognostic factor in breast cancer patients.

SENTINEL LYMPH NODE BIOPSY (SLNB)

Sentinel lymph node biopsy has revolutionised management of clinically node-negative breast cancer patients. The majority of studies validating the use of SLNB have restricted its use to T1 or T2 tumours. Larger tumours have a higher rate of ALN metastasis, and locally advanced tumour cells may infiltrate draining lymphatics, decreasing the identification rates of sentinel nodes and leading to an increased false negative ratio.[4] As such the American Society of Clinical Oncology (ASCO) guidelines have not recommended the use of SLNB for breast cancer patients with large or locally advanced tumours (T3 or T4).[5]

Where SLNB is performed, accuracy of surgeons in correctly identifying the sentinel node improves with experience, with a greater than 90 per cent rate of sentinel node identification and a false negative ratio of less than 5 per cent reported amongst surgeons having performed a minimum of 30 cases.[6] In the United Kingdom a national training programme has been initiated to standardise the technique of SLNB wherein a series of 30 cases is performed by the trainee surgeon. These procedures are then audited centrally to ensure the optimal performance of SLNB.[4]

Key Points

- Sentinel lymph node biopsy is possible in 96 per cent of cases and with a negative SLNB, SLN surgery without axillary lymph node dissection (ALND) is a safe and effective therapy for breast cancer patients
- Sentinel lymph node biopsy in the presence of palpable ALNs is not recommended.

Technique

Various techniques have been reported to identify the SLN, with both radioisotopes and blue dye used in the setting of breast cancer. A recent meta-analysis of 69 trials incorporating 8,059 patients comparing the differing techniques, reported accurate mapping of SLNs in 89.2 per cent of cases using radioisotopes, 83.1 per cent using blue dye and 91.9 per cent through combing both techniques.[7] Similarly false negatives were reduced to 7 per cent, when both techniques were used, leading the authors to recommend the combined use of blue dye and radioisotope to correctly identify the SLN.

Initial studies recommended the peri-tumoral injection of blue dye or radioisotope, however this has limited application in a clinically impalpable tumour. As such intra and sub-dermal injection of the skin above the tumour or peri and sub-areolar injection are possible sites for injection. A recent study reported comparable accuracy between peri-areolar and peri-tumoral injection in SLN detection. This was a prospective randomised controlled trial (RCT) consisting of 449 patients.[8] A further RCT of 400 breast cancers comparing intra-dermal, sub-areolar and intra-parenchymal injection of radioisotope reported the superiority of intra-dermal injection for SLN biopsy and mapping both in terms of increased frequency of localisation (95%) and decreased time to first localisation (mean 8 minutes).[9]

Removal of SLNs

Sentinel lymph nodes can be identified in approximately 96 per cent of cases with a low false negative ratio, with most surgeons identifying between one and three nodes.[10,11] A recent prospective study involving 803 cases to assess the upper threshold for the number of SLNs removed reported that metastasis was detected in the first four SLNs removed in 99.6 per cent of node-positive tumours, and as such removal of more than four nodes may be considered unnecessary.[12] Although removal of only one SLN minimises axillary morbidity and decreases operative time, it is associated with a false negative ratio of 10 per cent.[12] As such, some authors have suggested the removal of two to four SLNs for optimum staging.[4]

Key Points

- Sentinel lymph node biopsy in patients with ductal carcinoma in situ (DCIS) is not routinely recommended, but should be considered in patients with a palpable or mammographic mass or high grade dysplasia
- Completion ALN dissection remains the standard of care for patients with SNL involvement
- Routine level III axillary clearance in node positive patients is an acceptable standard of care in high-risk patients.

Prognostic Value of SLNB

Negative SLNB

The widespread application of SLNB spares many patients the potential side-effects of ALND such as lymphoedema without compromising the curative effect of surgery in patients with a negative SLNB.[13] Multi-institutional studies and prospective randomised controlled trials have demonstrated the safety of omitting ALND for breast cancer patients whose sentinel node is free of disease.[10,14,15] The largest of these, the NSABP B-32 trial assessed 5,611 women across 80 centres. This randomised controlled phase III trial reported that overall survival, disease-free survival and regional control were statistically comparable between groups, concluding that with a negative SLNB, SLN surgery without ALND is a safe and effective.[16]

Positive SLNB

Current guidelines, and most specialist surgeons, recommend ALND in breast cancer patients with a positive SLNB, however debate continues as to whether ALND should be routinely performed on all patients with tumour-involved SLNs on biopsy.

It has previously been reported that in 40 to 60 per cent of cases, the SLN has been the only lymph node involved by cancer, suggesting that a subsequent ALND offers little additional diagnostic or therapeutic benefit while carrying associated increased morbidity.[17] However a follow-up study of 4,008 procedures from Memorial Sloan-Kettering Cancer Centre in the USA demonstrated a significantly higher recurrence rate in SLNB positive patients not undergoing ALND (1.4% vs 0.18%, p=0.013), and a more recent meta-analysis recommended completion ALND for all SLNB positive cases having reported that 48.3 per cent of patients with a positive SLNB had non-SLN involvement.[7]

The American College of Surgeons Oncology Group (ACSOG) Z0011 randomised trial was recently published comparing sentinel lymph node dissection (SLND) with or without axillary dissection up to level II in patients with SLN metastases. Overall 891 patients were randomised, with a median of 17 ALNs removed in those undergoing axillary dissection compared with two nodes removed in those undergoing sentinel node dissection alone. Both groups of patients received whole breast irradiation and adjuvant systemic therapy. Despite those undergoing axillary dissection having significantly more positive lymph nodes removed there were no statistically significant differences in local recurrence or regional recurrence at a median follow-up of 6.2 years.[18] However, a limitation of this study is the low axillary tumour burden noted in the cohort of patients studied, due to reluctance at trial design stage to randomise patients with a high axillary burden and instead this cohort underwent ALND.

The prognostic significance of micrometastases within SLN remains unclear. A recent meta-analysis comprising of 25 studies and 789 patients reported a risk of non-SLN metastasis of 10 to 15 per cent in cases with SLN micrometastases.[1] However, whether the risk of up to 15 per cent of having tumour tissue remaining in the axilla is acceptable remains to be decided, particularly when we consider that a proportion of these patients with non-SLN involvement after a SLNB showing micrometastases may never suffer from their axillary metastases. Other variables such as patient age and tumour size must be considered when making the clinical decision about further axillary surgery. Similarly completion ALND for breast cancer patients with isolated tumour cells identified on immunohistochemistry is particularly controversial due to the low yield of additional positive ALNs. Despite this, with a SLNB revealing isolated tumour cells an ALND remains an acceptable management option.[5]

RADIOLOGICAL STAGING OF AXILLA

Surgical removal and the histopathological examination of ALNs is the most reliable and accurate way of staging of the axilla. However preoperative scintigraphic mapping combined with intra-operative probe detection is often used in SLN identification. Injection of ^{99m}Tc colloid allows for marking of the skin over each detected radioactive focus on subsequent scintigraphic images of the neck and chest.

By providing a map of the distribution of the radiotracer this could allow for more efficient identification of SLNs intraoperatively.[2,19] However previous trials have shown no significant benefit in routine preoperative lymphoscintigraphy for the identification of SLNs.[20] As such its routine use given the associated time and cost, as well as questionable therapeutic relevance of nonaxillary draining nodes identified remains controversial.

Other imaging techniques such as ultrasound or magnetic resonance mammography are insufficiently accurate alone in staging the axilla, particularly with tumour deposits less than 0.5 cm.[21] As such no radiological investigation at present is sufficient to obviate the need for formal axillary staging using SLNB or ALND. Although fluoro-deoxyglucose positron emission tomography/CT scan (FDG PET/CT) is extremely effective in detection of distant breast cancer metastasis with a specificity of 95 to 100 per cent, it is less sensitive than SLNB for detection of lymph node metastasis.[22] However it may have a future role in axillary node evaluation. As a single investigation, it's specificity is too low to replace SLNB for assessment in the short-term, however it may play a role in avoiding unnecessary SLNB in patients with nodal involvement detected on FDG PET/CT.[2]

Clinically Palpable ALNs

Clinically palpable ALNs detected preoperatively in breast cancer patients is widely held to be a contraindication to SLNB.[4] However ultrasound guided fine-needle aspiration (FNA) or core biopsy has been reported as yielding a positive result for only 41 per cent of axillae containing macrometastases,[23] and it has been previously reported that clinical examination of the axilla is falsely positive in up to 30 per cent of cases.[24] In fact, a recent prospective study of 2,027 consecutive SLNB procedures described a false positive clinical examination of the axilla rate of 53 per cent raising the question of whether SLNB should be considered in breast cancer patients with palpable ALNs and an indeterminate FNA or core biopsy using ultrasound.[25] Despite this, best practice guidelines relating to management of clinically palpable ALNs, recommend their removed irrespective of SLNB results.[5] As such SLNB in the presence of palpable lymph nodes cannot be recommended.

THERAPEUTIC MANAGEMENT OF THE AXILLA

Axillary Lymph Node Dissection (ALND)

Axillary clearance is associated with considerable morbidity and mortality and as such will always be a source of surgical controversy. The advent of SLNB has had a dramatic effect on reducing the proportion of patients undergoing axillary clearance, although still 20 to 30 per cent of patients who undergo SLNB will then subsequently be considered for an axillary clearance by virtue of their node positivity.[26]

ALN involvement has been proposed as a marker of tumour dissemination rather than a potential source of tumour dissemination itself. As such it has been suggested that axillary dissection is only a staging procedure and has no therapeutic role.[3] Despite this, a previous meta-analysis of six trials and almost 3,000 patients revealed a survival benefit of 5.4 per cent in patients undergoing prophylactic ALND.[27]

The ACOSOG Z0011 trial recently reported postoperative morbidity data on 891 patients, 445 of whom underwent SLNB alone with the remainder underwent SLNB with ALND. In patients undergoing SLNB with ALND, there was a significantly higher rate of surgical site infection, seroma and paraesthesia. In addition, the incidence of lymphoedema at 12 months follow-up was noted to be significantly increased in the group undergoing ALND (13% vs 2%, $p<0.001$).[28] When ALND is combined with axillary irradiation, the risk of lymphoedema may rise to 30 to 40 per cent.[29]

The axilla is divided into three levels, described in relation to the pectoralis minor muscle. Level I nodes lie up to the lateral border of the muscle, level II deep to the muscle, and level III nodes are located from above the medial border of the muscle to the apex of the axilla.

As discussed, an axillary clearance is an acceptable management option following a finding of SLN micro or macrometastases. However there exists considerable variation in the level of clearance surgeons perform for invasive breast cancer.[30]

Without adequate clearance of involved ALNs, recurrence rates have been reported as high as 18.6 per cent.[31] At present it is suggested that patients with SLN positive breast cancer undergo at least a level II clearance.[32] However a recent UK survey reported that 49 per cent of breast surgeons routinely perform level III clearances,[33] and worldwide there is considerable variance in the number of levels performed. It has been suggested that decisions as to which patients should undergo level III rather than level II clearance are likely to be based upon individual institutional policies rather than providing an individually tailored treatment regime.[26] The use of SLNB has added to this debate as patients undergoing ALND are at increased risk of level III involvement since they have been selected on the basis of proven ALN disease.

A recent Irish study of 2,850 patients, of whom 747 were SLN positive and undergoing ALND demonstrated involvement of level III in 19 per cent, with tumour size, extranodal invasion, lymphovascular invasion and lobular invasive disease significantly associated with level III involvement on multivariate analysis.[26] Indeed a study of patients with sentinel node micrometastases undergoing level III clearances demonstrated an 18 per cent rate of non-SLN involvement in the setting of SLN micrometastases, with 4 per cent of those involving level III.[30] In addition, recent evidence suggests that a clearance to level III as compared with level I/II does not necessarily increase morbidity, despite being associated with a longer operative time and greater intraoperative blood loss.[34] Overall the proportion of level III involvement in high-risk patients is considerable, and judicious planning is necessary in planning the extent of axillary surgery in patients with proven node positive disease on SLNB.

Key Point

- Recent evidence suggests that in patients with a low axillary tumour burden sentinel node dissection alone may have comparable survival rates to ALND.

Axillary Node Sampling (ANS)

An alternative approach to reducing the morbidity associated with ALND includes axillary node sampling. Introduced more than 30 years ago in the UK, using this technique at least four palpable lymph nodes need to be removed from the axillary tail and lower axillary fat to obtain 95 per cent accuracy in staging the axilla. Two previous RCT assessed ANS followed by axillary radiotherapy compared with ALND in breast cancer patients post-mastectomy.[35,36] In node negative patients, there was a significantly higher rate of axillary recurrence in those undergoing ANS alone compared with ALND (6.8% vs 1.6%, p=0.017), however overall long-term survival between both groups was comparable with a median follow-up of 10 years. In addition, in node positive patients, there was no significant difference in axillary recurrence between those undergoing ALND, and those undergoing ANS with subsequent irradiation. In terms of morbidity, although arm swelling was increased in those undergoing ALND, those undergoing ANS with radiotherapy reported decreased shoulder movement.

More recently a retrospective study of 381 patients compared ANS with ALND with a median follow-up of 6.5 years. No difference in axillary recurrence rates between the two groups was noted. Similarly overall survival was 84 per cent and comparable between both groups. With regard to complications and treatment toxicity, the incidence of lymphoedema was again higher in the group undergoing ALND compared to ANC and subsequent radiotherapy (16% vs 7%).

Overall a policy of selective ANS in combination with postoperative radiotherapy for breast cancer patients with node positive disease leads to comparable outcomes to patients undergoing ALND alone without a detrimental effect on long-term survival. However there remain criticisms regarding the procedure of ANS being too random and unpredictable.[4]

Management of the Axilla in DCIS

DCIS by definition has no invasive foci. However 10 to 29 per cent of patients initially diagnosed with DCIS on core biopsy are found to have a focus of invasive cancer at the time of definitive surgery. Nodal metastasis in DCIS is uncommon, occurring in only 0 to 3 per cent of cases; however a recent study of 398 patients with DCIS found that the presence of a palpable tumour was an independent predictor of a positive SLN.[37] Current data suggest that SLNB should not be routinely performed in the presence of DCIS, the possibility of SLNB should be discussed with younger patients, those diagnosed by core-needle biopsy, those with a high grade nuclear lesion, or those with a palpable or mammographic mass (>2.5 cm).[13,37,38]

RADIOTHERAPY AS TREATMENT OF AXILLARY DISEASE

Axillary radiotherapy for treatment of the axilla has been compared with ALND in a number of randomised controlled trials. In one such study of 1,851 breast cancer patients' comparison was made between axillary radiotherapy and ALND in post-mastectomy patients with node negative breast cancer.[31] Although axillary recurrence rates were higher in those receiving axillary radiation (3.1% vs 1.4%), there were no significant differences in overall survival at 10 years follow-up. A further prospective RCT reporting follow-up of 15 years between axillary radiotherapy and ALND in 658 node negative patients was recently published. The authors reported a significantly lower recurrence rate (1% vs 3%, p=0.04) in patients treated with ALND rather than radiotherapy alone. However there were no differences in recurrence rates in the breast or distal metastases, and long-term survival was comparable between both groups of patients.[39]

Patients with a positive SLN are generally treated with ALND. In 2001, the European Organisation of Research and Treatment of Cancer (EORTC) initiated the 10981 AMAROS trial, a phase III study comparing axillary radiotherapy with ALND in patients with node positive disease. Accrual of the necessary 4,767 patients is ongoing and estimated to be completed in 2010.[40]

Key Point

- Preliminary reports suggest that radiotherapy alone may be an effective strategy in treating involved axillary nodes with no decrease in overall survival when compared to traditional surgery.

CONCLUSION

Optimal management of the axilla is paramount in breast cancer patients, with several surgical approaches available to from both a diagnostic and therapeutic perspective. Axillary nodal status remains the most important prognostic factor for patients with breast cancer, and at present axillary surgery remains the most reliable method of staging the axilla, with SLNB an accurate staging procedure for early (T1-T2, cN0) invasive breast cancer.

Axillary lymph node dissection remains an acceptable management option for patients with SLN metastases with level III clearance an acceptable routine practice in high-risk patients. However recent evidence suggests that in patients with a low axillary tumour burden, treatment with breast conserving surgery and adjuvant systemic therapy may not be improved by ALND compared with sentinel node dissection alone. There is also some preliminary evidence to suggest that radiotherapy alone can be used effectively in treating involved ALNs with comparable long-term regional control and overall survival rates while avoiding axillary dissection. However further evidence is necessary to confirm this.

Key Points for Clinical Practice

- Axillary node involvement is the most important prognostic factor in breast cancer patients
- Sentinel lymph node biopsy is possible in 96 per cent of cases and with a negative SLNB, sentinel lymph node surgery without ALND is a safe and effective therapy for breast cancer patients
- Sentinel lymph node biopsy in the presence of palpable ALNs is not recommended
- Sentinel lymph node biopsy in patients with DCIS is not routinely recommended but should be considered in patients with a palpable or mammographic mass or high grade dysplasia
- Completion ALND remains the standard of care for patients with SLN involvement
- Routine level III axillary clearance in node positive patients is an acceptable standard of care in high-risk patients
- Recent evidence suggests that in patients with a low axillary tumour burden sentinel node dissection alone may have comparable survival rates to ALND
- Preliminary reports suggest that radiotherapy alone may be an effective strategy in treating involved axillary nodes with no decrease in overall survival when compared to traditional surgery.

REFERENCES

1. Cserni G, Gregori D, Merletti F, et al. Meta-analysis of non-sentinel node metastases associated with micrometastatic sentinel nodes in breast cancer. Br J Surg 2004;91(10):1245-52.

2. Cheng G, Kurita S, Torigian DA, et al. Current status of sentinel lymph-node biopsy in patients with breast cancer. Eur J Nucl Med Mol Imaging. 2011 Mar;38(3):562-75. Epub 2010 Aug 11.

3. Morton DL, Wen DR, Wong JH, et al. Technical details of intraoperative lymphatic mapping for early stage melanoma. Arch Surg 1992;127(4):392-9.

4. Samphao S, Eremin JM, El-Sheemy M, et al. Management of the axilla in women with breast cancer: current clinical practice and a new selective targeted approach. Ann Surg Oncol 2008;15(5):1282-96.

5. Lyman GH, Giuliano AE, Somerfield MR, et al. American Society of Clinical Oncology guideline recommendations for sentinel lymph node biopsy in early-stage breast cancer. J Clin Oncol 2005;23(30):7703-20.

6. de Mascarel I, Bonichon F, Coindre JM, et al. Prognostic significance of breast cancer axillary lymph node micrometastases assessed by two special techniques: reevaluation with longer follow-up. Br J Cancer 1992;66(3):523-7.

7. Kim T, Giuliano AE, Lyman GH. Lymphatic mapping and sentinel lymph node biopsy in early-stage breast carcinoma: a metaanalysis. Cancer 2006;106(1):4-16.

8. Rodier JF, Velten M, Wilt M, et al. Prospective multicentric randomized study comparing periareolar and peritumoral injection of radiotracer and blue dye for the detection of sentinel lymph node in breast sparing procedures: FRANSENODE trial. J Clin Oncol 2007;25(24):3664-9.

9. Povoski SP, Olsen JO, Young DC, et al. Prospective randomized clinical trial comparing intradermal, intraparenchymal, and subareolar injection routes for sentinel lymph node mapping and biopsy in breast cancer. Ann Surg Oncol 2006;13(11):1412-21.

10. Veronesi U, Paganelli G, Viale G, et al. Sentinel-lymph-node biopsy as a staging procedure in breast cancer: update of a randomised controlled study. Lancet Oncol 2006;7(12):983-90.

11. Goyal A, Newcombe RG, Chhabra A, et al. Factors affecting failed localisation and false-negative rates of sentinel node biopsy in breast cancer—results of the ALMANAC validation phase. Breast Cancer Res Treat 2006;99(2):203-8.

12. Goyal A, Newcombe RG, Mansel RE. Clinical relevance of multiple sentinel nodes in patients with breast cancer. Br J Surg 2005;92(4):438-42.

13. Purushotham AD, Upponi S, Klevesath MB, et al. Morbidity after sentinel lymph node biopsy in primary breast cancer: results from a randomized controlled trial. J Clin Oncol 2005;23(19):4312-21.

14. Gill PG. Sentinel lymph node biopsy versus axillary clearance in operable breast cancer: The RACS SNAC trial, a multicenter randomized trial of the Royal Australian College of Surgeons (RACS) Section of Breast Surgery, in collaboration with the National Health and Medical Research Council Clinical Trials Center. Ann Surg Oncol 2004;11(3 Suppl):216S-21S.

15. Mansel RE, Fallowfield L, Kissin M, et al. Randomized multicenter trial of sentinel node biopsy versus standard axillary treatment in operable breast cancer: the ALMANAC Trial. J Natl Cancer Inst 2006;98(9):599-609.

16. Krag DN, Anderson SJ, Julian TB, et al. Sentinel-lymph-node resection compared with conventional axillary-lymph-node dissection in clinically node-negative patients with breast cancer: overall survival findings from the NSABP B-32 randomised phase 3 trial. Lancet Oncol 2010;11(10):927-33.

17. Grube BJ, Giuliano AE. Modification of the sentinel node technique: it was a hit in New York, but will it play in Poughkeepsie? Ann Surg Oncol 2001;8(1):3-6.

18. Giuliano AE, McCall L, Beitsch P, et al. Locoregional recurrence after sentinel lymph node dissection with or without axillary dissection in patients with sentinel lymph node metastases: the American College of Surgeons Oncology Group Z0011 randomized trial. Ann Surg 2010;252(3):426-32.

19. Krag DN, Anderson SJ, Julian TB, et al. Technical outcomes of sentinel-lymph-node resection and conventional axillary-lymph-node dissection in patients with clinically node-negative breast cancer: results from the NSABP B-32 randomised phase III trial. Lancet Oncol 2007;8(10):881-8.

20. McMasters KM, Wong SL, Tuttle TM, et al. Preoperative lymphoscintigraphy for breast cancer does not improve the ability to identify axillary sentinel lymph nodes. Ann Surg 2000;231(5):724-31.

21. Patani NR, Dwek MV, Douek M. Predictors of axillary lymph node metastasis in breast cancer: a systematic review. Eur J Surg Oncol 2007;33(4):409-19.

22. Aukema TS, Straver ME, Peeters MJ, et al. Detection of extra-axillary lymph node involvement with FDG PET/CT in patients with stage II-III breast cancer. Eur J Cancer 2010;46(18):3205-10.

23. Deurloo EE, Tanis PJ, Gilhuijs KG, et al. Reduction in the number of sentinel lymph node procedures by preoperative ultrasonography of the axilla in breast cancer. Eur J Cancer 2003;39(8):1068-73.

24. Fisher B, Wolmark N, Bauer M, et al. The accuracy of clinical nodal staging and of limited axillary dissection as a determinant of histologic nodal status in carcinoma of the breast. Surg Gynecol Obstet 1981;152(6):765-72.

25. Specht MC, Fey JV, Borgen PI, et al. Is the clinically positive axilla in breast cancer really a contraindication to sentinel lymph node biopsy? J Am Coll Surg 2005;200(1):10-4.

26. Dillon MF, Advani V, Masterson C, et al. The value of level III clearance in patients with axillary and sentinel node positive breast cancer. Ann Surg 2009;249(5):834-9.

27. Orr RK. The impact of prophylactic axillary node dissection on breast cancer survival—a Bayesian meta-analysis. Ann Surg Oncol 1999;6(1):109-16.

28. Lucci A, McCall LM, Beitsch PD, et al. Surgical complications associated with sentinel lymph node dissection (SLND) plus axillary lymph node dissection compared with SLND alone in the American College of Surgeons Oncology Group Trial Z0011. J Clin Oncol 2007;25(24):3657-63.

29. Kunkler IH. Radiotherapy of the regional lymph nodes: shooting at the sheriff? Breast. 2009;18(Suppl 3):S112-20.

30. Dillon MF, Hayes BD, Quinn CM, et al. The Extent of Axillary Lymph Node Clearance Required Following Detection of Sentinel Node Micro-metastases. Breast J 2010 Jul 6. [Epub ahead of print]

31. Fisher B, Anderson S, Bryant J, et al. Twenty-year follow-up of a randomized trial comparing total mastectomy, lumpectomy, and lumpectomy plus irradiation for the treatment of invasive breast cancer. N Engl J Med 2002;347(16):1233-41.

32. NIH consensus conference. Treatment of early-stage breast cancer. JAMA 1991;265(3):391-5.

33. Gaston MS, Dixon JM. A survey of surgical management of the axilla in UK breast cancer patients. Eur J Cancer 2004;40(11):1738-42.

34. Kodama H, Nio Y, Iguchi C, et al. Ten-year follow-up results of a randomised controlled study comparing level-I vs level-III axillary lymph node dissection for primary breast cancer. Br J Cancer 2006;95(7):811-6.

35. Forrest AP, Everington D, McDonald CC, et al. The Edinburgh randomized trial of axillary sampling or clearance after mastectomy. Br J Surg 1995;82(11):1504-8.

36. Chetty U, Jack W, Prescott RJ, et al. Management of the axilla in operable breast cancer treated by breast conservation: a randomized clinical trial. Edinburgh Breast Unit. Br J Surg 2000;87(2):163-9.

37. Yen TW, Hunt KK, Ross MI, et al. Predictors of invasive breast cancer in patients with an initial diagnosis of ductal carcinoma in situ: a guide to selective use of sentinel lymph node biopsy in management of ductal carcinoma in situ. J Am Coll Surg 2005;200(4):516-26.

38. Meijnen P, Oldenburg HS, Loo CE, et al. Risk of invasion and axillary lymph node metastasis in ductal carcinoma in situ diagnosed by core-needle biopsy. Br J Surg 2007;94(8):952-6.

39. Louis-Sylvestre C, Clough K, Asselain B, et al. Axillary treatment in conservative management of operable breast cancer: dissection or radiotherapy? Results of a randomized study with 15 years of follow-up. J Clin Oncol 2004;22(1):97-101.

40. Straver ME, Meijnen P, van Tienhoven G, et al. Sentinel node identification rate and nodal involvement in the EORTC 10981-22023 AMAROS trial. Ann Surg Oncol 2010;17(7):1854-61.

SECTION FIVE

VASCULAR SURGERY

CHAPTER■ **THIRTEEN**

Recent Advances in Endovascular Management of Aortic Aneurysms

Jane Cross, Dominic Simring, Toby Richards

INTRODUCTION

Endovascular aneurysm repair (EVAR) has changed the management of aortic aneurysms. In this chapter, the author documents the chronological evidence for EVAR and details the following recent advances; abdominal aortic aneurysm (AAA) screening, the use of EVAR for ruptured aneurysms and development in branched and fenestrated EVAR.

Initially conceived as a treatment for patients unfit for open surgery, it was a decade after Parodi's[1] first case that EVAR emerged as a viable treatment option for infra-renal AAA (Figs 13.1A and B). Prototypes in the early 1990s were often 'home made' and predisposed to complications. Two registries launched in 1996 documented these learning curves [Registry for Endovascular Treatment of Aneurysms (UK) (RETA) and EUROSTAR from 14 European countries].

Early enthusiasm was tempered by poor proximal fixation, stent graft migration and delayed AAA rupture. By its closure in 2006 EUROSTAR produced data on 11,208 EVAR. This level two evidence influenced patient management.

Second generation graft designs and with RETA, provided methodology for two UK randomised endovascular aneurysm repair trials (EVAR I and II). Started in 1999, as the second generation devices became available, these trials combined with the Dutch Randomized Endovascular Aneurysm Management Trial (DREAM) produced level one evidence for EVAR in 2004 and 2005. From then onwards, the last five years has seen a steady expansion of EVAR use which is now regarded as standard management for AAA (Figs 13.2A to C).

The next generation infrarenal devices include modifications in graft flexibility and lower profile design to increase ease of use and applicability. Developments of fenestrated and branched graft design show recent advances in EVAR in complex AAA.

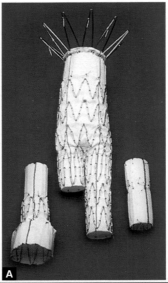

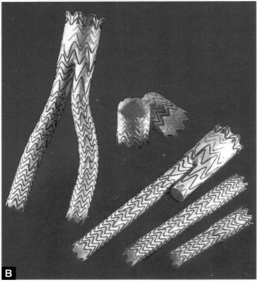

Figs 13.1A and B: Some commercially available modular infra-renal EVAR devices; (A) The Cook Zenith device. This is made up of three parts: a main body and two legs. The graft itself is made of polyester, and prolene suture is used to sew the graft material to a frame of stainless steel stents. The uncovered stents at proximal end are designed to sit above the renal arteries (supra-renal fixation).The graft has several gold markers to aid orientation; (B) The GORE Excluder device. The graft is made from polytetrafluoroethylene (PTFE) with outer self-expanding Nitinol stents

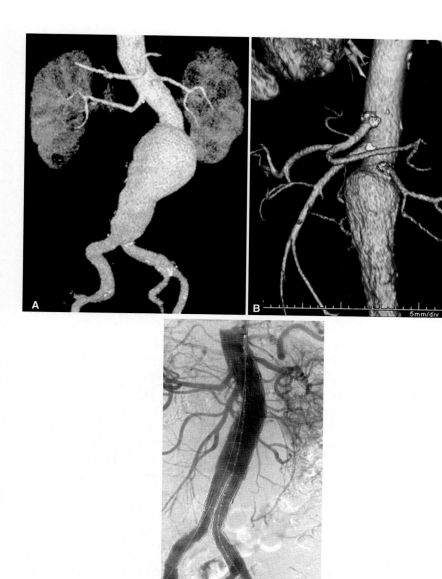

Figs 13.2A to C: (A) 3-D reconstruction of a CT angiogram showing an infrarenal aneurysm. The aortic neck, seen as a section of normal aorta below the renal arteries provide an adequate proximal landing zone for EVAR; (B) 3-D reconstruction of a CT angiogram showing an infrarenal aneurysm; however this patient has an inadequate neck length for a standard infra-renal device as the aneurysm can be seen to arise immediately below the renal arteries; (C) Completion of angiography following infra-renal EVAR

LEVEL ONE EVIDENCE FOR EVAR

EVAR I and II[2] Trial Design

Between September 1999 and December 2003 patients aged over 60, with an AAA greater than 5.5 cm, anatomically suitable for EVAR were included in two randomised trials. EVAR I comprised patients considered fit for open repair and EVAR II contained those, which were considered unfit for the repair. Forty one centres were eligible as defined by completion of 20 previous cases (entered to RETA). EVAR I randomly allocated patients to open or endovascular repair whereas EVAR II compared EVAR with conservative management. Primary outcome in both the trials was all cause mortality. Secondary outcomes were aneurysm related mortality, postoperative complications, secondary interventions, quality of life scores and cost effectiveness.

DREAM[3] Trial Design

Between November 2000 and December 2003 patients with AAA greater than 5 cm and anatomically suitable for EVAR were included in a randomised trial if deemed fit for open surgery as defined by a cardiologist/internalist. As with EVAR I, EVAR was compared to open surgery. There were 26 participating centres in Holland and four in Belgium. Teams had performed at least five EVAR and were proctored until they had performed 20. Primary endpoints were operative mortality and morbidity, secondary endpoints and additional assessments were event free survival, quality of life, length of hospital stay and costs. Each complication was assessed by an independent blinded assessor.

EVAR I[4] Early Results

These were reported in 2004 on patients recruited by December 31st 2003. Of all screened individuals 54 per cent of were anatomically suitable for EVAR. A total of 1,082 patients were randomised in EVAR Trial 1, 543 allocated EVAR and 539 allocated open repair. Demographic profiles were similar. The 30-day mortality was lower in the EVAR group, 1.7 per cent (9/531) *versus* 4.7 per cent (24/516) in the open group [odds ratio 0.35 (95% CI 0.16-0.77) P=0.009]. Secondary interventions were more common in patients allocated to EVAR (9.8% *versus* 5.8%, P=0.02).

DREAM[5] Early Results

DREAM also reported in 2004 with 351 patients randomised, 174 to open repair and 171 patients EVAR. Patient demographics were similar. The 30-day mortality was again lower in the EVAR group, 1.2 per cent (2/171) *versus* 4.6 per cent (8/174) for open repair [risk ratio 3.9 (95% CI 0.9 to

32.9, P=0.10)]. The combined rates of operative mortality and severe complications were 4.7 per cent (8/171) in EVAR and 9.8 per cent (17/174) in open repair [risk ratio 2.1 (95% CI 0.9 to 5.4, P=0.10)]. EVAR was associated with shorter duration of surgery, less blood loss and blood replacement, less postoperative respiratory ventilation, less change in haematocrit, shorter ITU/HDU stay and shorter hospital stay than open repair.

Publication of these trials in 2004 provided level one evidence for reduced early mortality from EVAR compared to open repair. DREAM was not statistically significant, due to low numbers (a third that of EVAR I). One reason suggested was withdrawal of funding for DREAM, as EVAR I had recruited and outcomes looked similar. These early results were augmented in 2005 with publication of EVAR I midterm results and those from EVAR II. Together they were a turning point in EVAR use. Although the first commercially available device was launched in 1999, it was not until publication of EVAR I and DREAM results that most vascular surgeons took EVAR as a valid alternative to open repair.

The UK National Vascular Database[6] report in 2004 did not report EVAR in the management of 3,444 AAA. In 2008, 1,580 EVAR were reported in 3,614 AAA (44%). Leading manufacturers have seen over 100,000 of their second generation devices deployed.

EVAR 1[7] Midterm Results

EVAR 1 reported four year outcomes. Overall at a median follow-up of 2.9 years 209 of 1,082 patients had died, 53 from aneurysm-related causes. Primary outcome of all-cause mortality was similar in both groups (about 28% P=0.46). Secondary outcome of aneurysm-related death was reduced following EVAR (4% *versus* 7%, P=0.04). Complications were more common following EVAR (41% *versus* 9% for open, P=0.04). Re-intervention occurred in 15 per cent following EVAR and 7 per cent of open repairs. 14 patients in the EVAR group were converted to open, 6 early and 8 late. Midterm results also reported improved initial quality of life scores following EVAR at three months with no differences seen after 12 months. EVAR was associated with increased costs of £13,257 versus £9,946 for the open repair group.

EVAR Trial 2[8]

338 patients were entered by December 31st 2003, 166 were allocated EVAR. Demographic profiles of the groups were similar. Fourteen patients died before intervention (six ruptured), 146 underwent EVAR (90%), four had open repair (2 for rupture), two were managed conservatively. Of 150 patients the median time from randomisation to surgery was 57 days. Of 172 patients randomised to no intervention, 125 (73%) adhered to

protocol, 47 crossed over (35 EVAR and 12 open repair). On intention to treat, 30 day EVAR group mortality was 9 per cent (n=13/150).

At four years 64 per cent of patients had died (n=142), 42 (30%) of these from aneurysm-related causes. There was no significant difference between the EVAR group and the no-intervention group for all cause mortality (HR1.21, P=0.25) or for aneurysm related mortality. Post hoc per protocol analysis showed no difference in all cause mortality (HR 1.07 P=0.7) or aneurysm related mortality (HR 0.77 P=0.43). Quality of Life had no difference between the groups and EVAR more expensive (£13,632 vs £4,983).

Outcomes of EVAR I and II cemented the early benefit for EVAR in 'fit patients' and clarified indications for EVAR in those 'unfit'. Criticisms of EVAR included the high rates of re-intervention, the need for long term surveillance and increased costs. Re-intervention was high, but reflected treatment of type II endoleaks. These are now regarded as benign, the majority resolving over six months and requiring re-intervention in the minority of cases. Costs have fallen with increasing use of duplex instead of CT for follow up, reduced hospital stay (median six days in EVAR I) and reduction in device costs. EVAR II had methodological criticisms on delay to treatment and large number of cross over cases between groups. Nevertheless post hoc analysis showed no advantage from EVAR. Early mortality in EVAR II was very high, significantly more than EVAR I perhaps suggesting poor patient selection; patients with very limited life expectancy. Definition by what is 'unfit' was confused by functional results (cardiac and lung function) that overlapped with those regarded 'fit' in EVAR I.

The EVAR trials demonstrated that doctors can effectively identify those patients in whom EVAR is not appropriate and in those appropriate, there was a better early outcome with reduced AAA related mortality.

Long-Term Results for EVAR 1 Trial[9]

In total 1,252 patients were recruited by 31st August 2004, 626 assigned to each group. Patients were followed up for a minimum of five years (mean 6 years, max 10 years). Of 524 deaths, 76 were aneurysm related. The 30 day mortality remained improved for EVAR [1.8% (11/614) *versus* 4.3% (26/602); P=0.02]. Although the endovascular group had an early benefit in terms of aneurysm related mortality, by the end of the study there was no difference between groups (P=0.73). There was no difference in all cause mortality (P=0.72). Complications were higher following EVAR (45.0% *versus* 12.4%; P=0.01). Re-intervention was also higher following EVAR (23.1% *versus* 8.8%; P=0.001). By the end of the study, 18 EVAR patients had been converted to open repair and delayed rupture following EVAR had occurred in 25 patients of whom 17 died.

Long-Term Results for EVAR 2 Trial[10]

In total 404 patients were recruited by 31st August 2004, 197 to EVAR and 207 to no intervention. During follow-up, median 3.1 years, 305 deaths occurred, 78 of which were aneurysm related. Primary endpoint of all cause mortality did not differ (P=0.97). Aneurysm related mortality was reduced with EVAR (P=0.02) despite a 30 day operative mortality of 7.3% (n=13). Overall the rate of aneurysm rupture in the no-intervention group was 12.4 per 100 person years. 70 patients in the no intervention group crossed over to the intervention group. During eight years of follow-up the average cost difference between each group was £9,826.

Key Points

- EVAR 1 demonstrated an improved short-term aneurysm related mortality, however by six years there was no difference and the long term results showed no benefit in either all cause or aneurysm related mortality
- EVAR 2 demonstrated no improvement in all cause mortality but long-term did show some benefit for aneurysm related mortality, however the all-cause mortality for these patients was very high.

Long-Term Results for DREAM Trial[11]

The median follow-up was 6.4 years and all patients were followed-up for a minimum of 5 years. There was no difference in overall survival (69.9% for open repair and 68.9% for EVAR, P=0.97). Aneurysm related mortality was not reported. The cumulative rates of freedom from secondary interventions were 81.9% for open repair and 70.4% for endovascular repair (95% Cl, 2.0 to 21.0; P = 0.03). Incisional hernia repair was the commonest intervention in the open group and endoleak or graft migration in the EVAR group.

Despite the results from these trials showing no long-term benefit from EVAR there has been little influence on current practise in the UK. Following early and mid term results in 2004 and 2005, there was a significant rise in EVAR use throughout the UK. EVAR offered reduced postoperative mortality. EVAR II suggested futility of offering elective intervention to unfit patients, a practise that has been adopted with conservative management for those with significant co-morbidities likely to live less than two to three years. However, EVAR is now firmly established in the management of AAA. For patients, able to attend follow-up with anatomically suitable AAA, EVAR is now the preferred first line treatment.

ANEURYSM SCREENING

Ruptured AAA accounts for about 6,000 deaths per year in England and Wales; 2 per cent of all deaths in men over the age of 65 years.

Between January 1997 and May 1999, the Multicentre Aneurysm Screening Study[12] (MASS) identified men aged 65 to 74 from four UK centres. 67,800 men were randomised, 33,839 invited for screening and 27,147 (80% of the invited group) men were scanned. 1,333 aneurysms (4.9% of patients scanned) were detected (defined as > 3 cm). Elective AAA repair was performed on 322 scanned patients and 92 in the control group. Primary endpoint showed 42 per cent reduction in aneurysm related mortality from screening (P=0.0002). Overall cost was £ 2.2 m, £ 63.39 per patient (95% confidence interval £ 53.31 to £ 73.48). Over four years the mean incremental cost effectiveness ratio for screening was £ 28 400 (£ 15 000 to £ 146 000) per life year gained, equivalent to about £ 36 000 per quality adjusted life year. After 10 years this figure is estimated to fall to around £ 8,000 per life year gained.

UK national screening was recommended. To date approximately one-third of regions in the UK are up and running. By March 2013, aneurysm screening is expected to be offered to all men in England.

Key Point

- Following the results of the MASS aneurysm screening study, a UK national screening programme has been started and will be nationwide by March 2013.

EVAR FOR RUPTURED ANEURYSMS

In 1994, Veith performed the first successful US EVAR for a ruptured AAA in a Jehovah's witness, at the same time Hopkinson reported a similar case in the UK.[13] Single centre series have reported mortality for REVAR (rupture treated by EVAR) of 17 to 24%[14,15] and two multicentre studies reported similar results of 26–45 per cent mortality[16,17] (Figure 13.3A to C).

In 2009, the UK National Vascular Database reported a RAAA open mortality of 38 per cent. A systematic review suggested REVAR was associated with reduced mortality (odds ratio 0.624).[18] Further REVAR was associated with lower postoperative physiological complications, reduced ITU and hospital stay compared to open repair.[16,18]

The VASCUNET multi-national database in 2008 reported 7,466 RAAA of which 6,468 were managed by open repair and only 478 by EVAR. Open mortality rate was 33 per cent compared to 15 per cent for EVAR. However, these data reflect selection bias. EVAR may be offered to more stable patients and those anatomically unsuitable for EVAR may present a more challenging

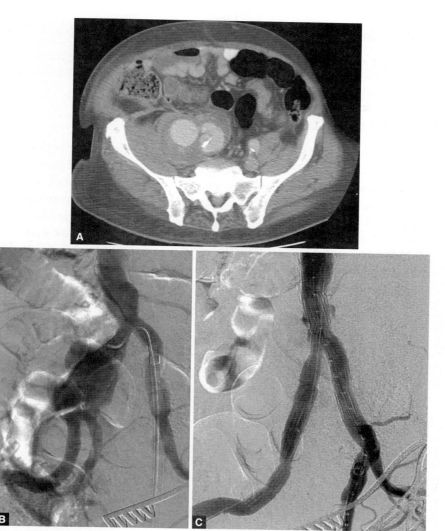

Figs 13.3A to C: (A) CT angiogram showing ruptured right common iliac artery. This patient presented with a 10 day history of urinary tract sepsis and sudden onset flank pain. Blood cultures showed *Salmonella*; (B) On table angiogram confirms normal aorta and aneurysm of right common iliac artery; (C) Following coiling of the right internal iliac artery an infra-renal EVAR was placed with extension into the right external iliac artery. The patient was discharged to home after five days on three months antibiotics. Follow-up at three years was normal

open repair. Previous randomised trials were terminated early due to lack of funding. Recruitment for the Immediate Management of the Patient with Ruptured aneurysm: Open Versus Endovascular repair trial (IMPROVE) started in October 2009.[19] The aim is to compare 600 patients, with a clinical diagnosis of RAAA, randomised to immediate CT scan and EVAR, or open repair with CT scan being optional. The trial is powered to show 14 per cent survival benefit for EVAR, projected recruitment is until 2014.

191

EVAR FOR SMALL ANEURYSMS

The UK small aneurysm trial[20] (UKSAT) and Aneurysm Detection and Management[21] (ADAM) trial showed no long-term survival benefit for early open surgery in patients with small (4.0–5.5 cm) symptomless AAA. These data have set the benchmark for AAA intervention over the last decade but results from EVAR have questioned this, since, there is a lower mortality rate from intervention, smaller AAA are more likely to be anatomically suitable for EVAR[22] and that in long-term follow up the majority of small AAA underwent intervention.[23] Two trials were undertaken to asses the role of EVAR for small AAA; Comparison of surveillance versus Aortic Endografting for Small Aneurysm Repair trial (CAESAR)[24] and Positive Impact of EndoVascular Options for Treating Aneurysms earLy (PIVOTAL)[25,26] trial.

CAESAR randomised 360 patients between 2004 and 2008 with 4.1 to 5.4 cm AAA to early EVAR (n=182) or surveillance and repair at a defined threshold (diameter ≥ 5.5 cm, enlargement >1 cm/year, symptoms) (n=178). Primary endpoint of all cause mortality showed no difference (P=0.6) at 54 months. Aneurysm related mortality, aneurysm rupture and major morbidity rates were similar.

PIVOTAL was a prospective 70 site trial of patients aged 40 to 90, morphologically suitable for EVAR with low risk co-morbidities, randomised to early EVAR *versus* surveillance for aneurysms 4 to 5cm in diameter. Of 728 patients, with a mean diameter of 4.5 cm, 362 were randomised to surveillance and 326 patients underwent intervention (EVAR n=322 and open repair n=4), although 112 patients assigned to surveillance underwent intervention (109 EVAR, 3 open). Primary endpoint of all cause mortality showed no difference at 20 months with 15 deaths in each group (4.1%) [HR for mortality in the early EVAR group was 1.01 (P=0.98)]. Other endpoints, rates were similar.

These trials suggested that EVAR could be undertaken in patients with small aneurysms but there was no benefit compared to surveillance in the endpoints assessed. Risk of rupture was lower than predicted in surveillance giving no advantage to EVAR. PIVOTAL was stopped early because of this. Debate on whether small AAA may grow out of anatomical suitability for EVAR was assessed in 221 patients under surveillance.[22] Smaller AAA were more likely to be anatomically suitable for EVAR, 76 per cent at mean 52 ± 9 mm, but rate of suitability did not decrease until the aneurysm measured 57 mm by CT scanning. These data imply that waiting until the aneurysm reaches 5.5 cm does not result in loss of suitability for EVAR. Any benefit from early intervention in small AAA is also affected by patient co-morbidities. 40 per cent of those followed up in the UKSAT died from other causes. Further optimal risk factor management with statins and ACE inhibitors may also slow AAA progression and delay rupture.

Key Point

- The CAESAR and PIVOTOL trials have shown no benefit to early EVAR in small aneurysms.

BRANCHED/FENESTRATED EVAR

The key principle to successful EVAR is to achieve an effective seal between the implanted stent graft and the native vessel. Guidelines for proximal landing zone suggest a neck greater than 15 mm, with angulation less than 60° that is not conical, without calcium or thrombus. Recent grafts have marginally extended these; neck greater than 10 mm that is straight or angulation less than 90° where the neck is more than 20 mm. Currently 25 to 50 per cent of all AAA remain unsuitable for standard EVAR including those juxtarenal, thoracoabdominal and iliac artery aneurysms. Development of fenestrations (holes) (Figs 13.4A to C) and branches (Figs 13.5A and B) in endograft design allows flow to aortic branch arteries through bridging stents. The use of fenestrated grafts (FEVAR) was first described in 1996.[27] Since then, over 4,000 cases have been undertaken in every section of the aorta. Grafts are custom made, specific to individual patient anatomy and can be technically challenging to insert. Outcome data is limited with only case series published.[28-34]

Fenestrated Endovascular Aneurysm Repair: World Wide Experience

Anderson[35] first published the proof of principle paper from Australia describing 13 patients (Aug 1998–May 2000) undergoing FEVAR. In the United States, two centres are licensed for complex EVAR. Cleveland has the largest FEVAR worldwide experience with 119 patients reported.[30] In Europe several case series have been reported, often with a mix of indications and devices. Chisci, et al. reported their centres' selected outcomes in patients undergoing open repair, off license infrarenal EVAR or if high risk FEVAR.[36] However, no trial has been undertaken to compare complex EVAR with open repair.

Nordon, et al[37] reviewed FEVAR (8 studies, n=368 patients) with historical open repair (12 studies, n=1164 patients), finding a 1.4 per cent

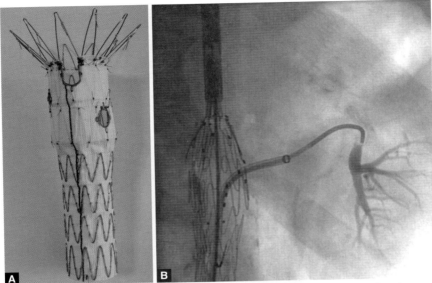

Figs 13.4A and B: Fenestrated endograft (FEVAR). Note the fenestrations for the renal arteries at the side and scallop for the superior mesenteric artery. This is a bespoke graft made to accommodate the individual anatomy of the intended patient. Note also the gold markers around the fenestrations and scallop to aid orientation; (B)FEVAR in situ. The main endograft is aligned and deployed. The top cap has not been deployed to maintain some manoeuvrability during target vessel cannulation. The target vessel (seen here the renal artery) is then cannulated through the endograft. Note the dots seen at the point. The catheter passes through the graft; these are the gold markers marking the edges of the fenestrations

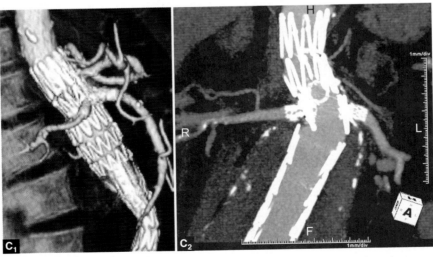

Fig. 13.4C: Completion CT angiogram showing the main endograft with bridging stents into target vessel

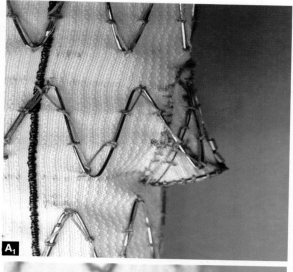

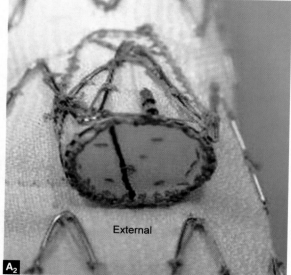

External

Fig. 13.5A: Branched endograft

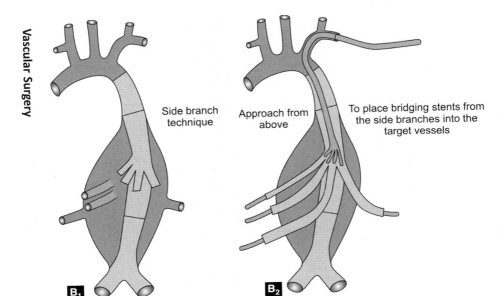

Fig. 13.5B: The device is inserted into position in the aorta. The picture illustrates the need for branches in larger and more proximal aneurysms. Fenestrations are only used when the aortic wall is closely opposed to the graft. With branched grafts, the target vessels are cannulated by accessing the brachial/subclavian artery and then passing the catheters in an antegrade direction from above

versus 3.6 per cent 30 day mortality in favour of FEVAR. The Ontario Health Technology[38] compared 5 FEVAR studies with 7 open studies giving a 1.8 per cent *versus* 3.1 per cent 30 day mortality in favour of FEVAR and a 12.8 per cent *versus* 23.7 per cent late mortality in favour of FEVAR. A recent review from Greece[39] of both fenestrated and branched grafts included 7 studies with a total of 155 patients. The majority of which were Crawford type IV aneurysms and they excluded "juxtarenal" aneurysms. They found a 7.1 per cent 30 day mortality for complex EVAR.

These data reflect selection bias and development of an emerging technology. Many cases were undertaken in patients deemed 'unfit' for open repair, reflecting a similar approach to when EVAR started. Reviewing the case series published, the author's contacted all authors identifying 10 studies with a total of 631 unduplicated patients. Patient demographics and indications were heterogeneous. Procedural endpoints included; operation times (median 180–375 min), fluoroscopy times (median 26–111 min) and target vessel cannulation (Table 13.1). Overall target vessel perfusion rates ranging from 90.5 to 100 per cent were reported in six papers, with failure of target vessel cannulation in 21 vessels (3.0%). There were three reports of intraoperative kidney loss, and six segmental renal infarcts were shown but none of these showed renal impairment. The length of hospital stay was reported in six papers (median 4–9 days). There were 11 deaths within 30 days, giving a 30 day mortality rate of 1.7 per cent. During follow-up there were a further 88 deaths (median 12–25, mode 24 months). Of these, six were aneurysm related deaths. Reports on late morbidity include loss of 50 target vessels, 10 stent fractures and 1 distraction of the modular components. 81 patients developed some post operative renal dysfunction, which was permanent in 53 patients. 10 patients required temporary renal support and 8 required permanent dialysis.

The reviews have highlighted the lack of evidence surrounding B/FEVAR, particularly in relation to open surgery and the problems involved in introducing a new technology.

The indications for the use of FEVAR are not clear and unit policies vary. The British Society of Endovascular Therapy (BSET) has recently published a consensus statement regarding the indications for FEVAR. It was generally agreed that FEVAR was not suitable for elderly frail high risk patients. However, there was a large area of equipoise regarding the use of FEVAR, particularly in young patients and those with short neck/juxtarenal aneurysms. Previous national registries have provided vital evidence for EVAR outcomes and have been used to set up formal trials. BSET has recently launched a national registry for B/FEVAR which may be the forerunner to a trial comparing endovascular repair to open repair of the complex aneurysm and to further define the indications for these modalities.

Key Point

- The evidence and indications for fenestrated and branched endografts is unclear and although current case series give a 1.7 per cent 30 day mortality.

Device Improvements

Diameter reducing ties allow for easier graft manipulation when there is a narrow segment in the visceral aorta and hold the graft away from the aortic wall aiding cannulation. Preloaded wires (threaded through the fenestrations at the time of manufacture) allow rapid passage of catheters directly to the fenestration or branch. Reduced delivery system size and greater sheath flexibility allow easier iliac access, reducing the need for iliac conduits.

Emerging device advances include "off-the-shelf" availability of fenestrated and branched endografts. Despite anatomical variation, the majority of renal arteries lie within a predictable region that can be accessed by pivoting fenestrations, rendering them suitable for pre-fabricated endografts in greater than 80 per cent of cases.[40] For more

TABLE 13.1

Numbers of scallops and fenestrations in the published series

Centre	RRA		LRA		SMA		Coeilac		Combined total
	S	F	S	F	S	F	S	F	
Groningen/Utrect	17	80	10	85	74	4	5	0	169F and 106 S
WA - Australia	25cb	66cb	0	10	21	3	0	1	70F and 46S
South Australia	0	14	0	ND	0	9	ND	ND	33F
France	ND	ND	ND	ND	ND	ND	ND	ND	269 F and 133 S
Malmo - Sweden	ND	ND	ND	ND	ND	ND	ND	ND	91 F and 133 S
Cleveland Ohio - US	231	L&R	L&R		76cb		0	1	308 cb
US	10	47	L&R		20	0	0	0	47F and 30S
Germany	24cb	64cb			10	12	7	2	78F and 41S
Liverpool - UK	10cb	68cb			28	7	1	1	76F and 29 S
St Mary's, London -UK	1	13	0	16	5	8	4	1	38F and 10S

RRA: right renal artery, S: scallop, F: fenestration, LRA: left renal artery, SMA: superior mesenteric artery, Cb: combined, ND: not documented

Increased number of fenestrations lead to longer operation times and increase the risk of complications such as failure of cannulation and target vessel loss. As shown, many series grouped fenestration numbers together making extrapolation between fenestration number and outcome difficult. The ratio of double: triple fenestrations between units was not uniform indicating potential differences in graft planning policies and design.

extensive aneurysms, pre-fabricated branched endografts have been demonstrated to be effective in a large proportion of cases. These "off-the-shelf" devices avoid the delay in manufacturing custom-made devices and will reduce cost.

CONCLUSION

EVAR has changed management of AAA in the last five years. EVAR is associated with shorter operation time, decreased blood loss, reduced hospital stay and improved 30 day operative mortality. Although, level one evidence supports EVAR for infrarenal AAA recent advances in graft technology are ahead of published evidence. Nevertheless, EVAR is emerging as the lead option for all aneurysm repairs.

Key Points for Clinical Practice

- EVAR 1 demonstrated an improved short-term aneurysm related mortality, however by six years, there was no difference and the long term results showed no benefit in either all cause or aneurysm related mortality
- EVAR 2 demonstrated no improvement in all cause mortality but long-term did show some benefit for aneurysm related mortality, however, the all cause mortality for these patients was very high
- The IMPROVE trial is a randomised control trial, now recruiting to determine the benefit of EVAR over open repair for ruptured abdominal aortic aneurysms
- The evidence and indications for fenestrated and branched endografts is unclear and although current case series give a 1.7 per cent 30 day mortality
- The CAESAR and PIVOTOL trials have shown no benefit to early EVAR in small aneurysms
- Following the results of the MASS aneurysm screening study, a UK national screening programme has been started and will be nationwide by March 2013.

REFERENCES

1. Parodi JC, Palmaz HD. Barone. Transfemoral intraluminal graft implantation for abdominal aortic aneurysms. Ann Vasc Surg 1991;5(6):491-9.
2. Brown LC, Epstein D, Manca A, et al. The UK Endovascular Aneurysm Repair (EVAR) trials: design, methodology and progress. Eur J Vasc Endovasc Surg 2004;27(4):372-81.
3. Prinssen ME, Buskens JD, Blankensteijn. The Dutch Randomised Endovascular Aneurysm Management (DREAM) trial. Background, design and methods. J Cardiovasc Surg 2002;43(3):379-84.
4. Greenhalgh RM, Brown LC, Kwong GP, et al. Comparison of endovascular aneurysm repair with open repair in patients with abdominal aortic

aneurysm (EVAR trial 1), 30-day operative mortality results: randomised controlled trial. Lancet. 2004;364(9437):843-8.

5. Prinssen M, Verhoeven EL, Buth J, et al. A randomized trial comparing conventional and endovascular repair of abdominal aortic aneurysms. N Engl J Med. 2004;351(16):1607-18.

6. Ireland, T.V.S.O.G.B.a., Fourth National Database Report 2004, in Dendrite clinical systems, Henley-upon-Thames. 2005.

7. Endovascular aneurysm repair versus open repair in patients with abdominal aortic aneurysm (EVAR trial 1): randomised controlled trial. Lancet. 2005;365(9478):2179-86.

8. Endovascular aneurysm repair and outcome in patients unfit for open repair of abdominal aortic aneurysm (EVAR trial 2): randomised controlled trial. Lancet. 2005;365(9478):2187-92.

9. United Kingdom EVAR Trial Investigators, Greenhalgh RM, Brown LC, et al. Endovascular versus open repair of abdominal aortic aneurysm. N Engl J Med. 2010;362(20):1863-71.

10. United Kingdom EVAR Trial Investigators, Greenhalgh RM, Brown LC, et al. Endovascular repair of aortic aneurysm in patients physically ineligible for open repair. N Engl J Med 2010;362(20):1872-80.

11. De Bruin JL, Baas AF, Buth J, et al. Long-term outcome of open or endovascular repair of abdominal aortic aneurysm. N Engl J Med 2010;362(20):1881-9.

12. Ashton HA, Buxton MJ, Day NE, et al. The Multicentre Aneurysm Screening Study (MASS) into the effect of abdominal aortic aneurysm screening on mortality in men: a randomised controlled trial. Lancet 2002;360(9345):1531-9.

13. Yusuf SW, Whitaker SC, Chuter TA, et al. Emergency endovascular repair of leaking aortic aneurysm. Lancet 1994;344(8937):1645.

14. Kubin K, Sodeck GH, Teufelsbauer H, et al. Endovascular therapy of ruptured abdominal aortic aneurysm: mid- and long-term results. Cardiovasc Intervent Radiol 2008;31(3):496-503.

15. Alsac JM, Desgranges P, Kobeiter H, et al. Emergency endovascular repair for ruptured abdominal aortic aneurysms: feasibility and comparison of early results with conventional open repair. Eur J Vasc Endovasc Surg 2005;30(6):632-9.

16. Silverberg D, Baril DT, Ellozy SH, et al. An 8-year experience with type II endoleaks: natural history suggests selective intervention is a safe approach. J Vasc Surg 2006;44(3):453-9.

17. Peppelenbosch N, Endograft treatment of ruptured abdominal aortic aneurysms using the Talent aortouniiliac system: an international multicenter study. J Vasc Surg 2006;43(6):1111-23.

18. Sadat U, Boyle JR, Walsh SR, et al. Endovascular vs open repair of acute abdominal aortic aneurysms—a systematic review and meta-analysis. J Vasc Surg 2008;48(1):227-36.

19. IMPROVE Trial, Powell JT, Thompson SG, et al. The Immediate Management of the Patient with Rupture: open Versus Endovascular repair (IMPROVE) aneurysm trial—ISRCTN 48334791 IMPROVE trialists. Acta Chir Belg 2009;109(6):678-80.

20. Powell JT, Greenhalgh RM, Ruckley CV, et al. The UK Small Aneurysm Trial. Ann N Y Acad Sci 1996;800:249-51.

21. Lederle FA, Johnson GR, Wilson SE, et al. The aneurysm detection and management study screening program: validation cohort and final results. Aneurysm Detection and Management Veterans Affairs Cooperative Study Investigators. Arch Intern Med 2000;160(10):1425-30.

22. Keefer A, Hislop S, Singh MJ, et al. The influence of aneurysm size on anatomic suitability for endovascular repair. J Vasc Surg 2010;52(4):873-7.

23. Powell JT, Brown LC, Forbes JF, et al. Final 12-year follow-up of surgery versus surveillance in the UK Small Aneurysm Trial. Br J Surg 2007;94(6):702-8.

24. Cao P, De Rango P, Verzini F, et al. Comparison of Surveillance Versus Aortic Endografting for Small Aneurysm Repair (CAESAR): results from a Randomised Trial. Eur J Vasc Endovasc Surg 2010.

25. Ouriel K. The PIVOTAL study: a randomized comparison of endovascular repair versus surveillance in patients with smaller abdominal aortic aneurysms. J Vasc Surg 2009;49(1):266-9.

26. Ouriel K, Clair DG, Kent KC, et al. Endovascular repair compared with surveillance for patients with small abdominal aortic aneurysms. J Vasc Surg 2010;51(5):1081-7.

27. Park JH, Chung JW, Choo IW, et al. Fenestrated stent-grafts for preserving visceral arterial branches in the treatment of abdominal aortic aneurysms: preliminary experience. J Vasc Interv Radiol 1996;7(6):819-23.

28. Amiot S, Haulon S, Becquemin JP, et al. Fenestrated endovascular grafting: the French multicentre experience. Eur J Vasc Endovasc Surg 2010;39(5):537-44.

29. Kristmundsson T. Fenestrated endovascular repair for juxtarenal aortic pathology. J Vasc Surg 2009;49(3):568-74.

30. O'Neill S, Greenberg RK, Haddad F, et al. A prospective analysis of fenestrated endovascular grafting: intermediate-term outcomes. Eur J Vasc Endovasc Surg 2006;32(2):115-23.

31. Ziegler P, Avgerinos ED, Umscheid T, et al. Fenestrated endografting for aortic aneurysm repair: a 7-year experience. J Endovasc Ther 2007;14(5):609-18.

32. Scurr JR, Brennan JA, Gilling-Smith GL, et al. Fenestrated endovascular repair for juxtarenal aortic aneurysm. Br J Surg 2008;95(3):326-32.

33. Bicknell CD, Cheshire NJ, Riga CV, et al. Treatment of complex aneurysmal disease with fenestrated and branched stent grafts. Eur J Vasc Endovasc Surg 2009;37(2):175-81.

34. Greenberg RK. Intermediate results of a United States multicenter trial of fenestrated endograft repair for juxtarenal abdominal aortic aneurysms. J Vasc Surg 2009;50(4):730-7.

35. Anderson JL, Berce M, Hartley DE. Endoluminal aortic grafting with renal and superior mesenteric artery incorporation by graft fenestration. J Endovasc Ther 2001;8(1):3-15.

36. Chisci E, Kristmundsson T, de Donato G, et al. The AAA with a challenging neck: outcome of open versus endovascular repair with standard and fenestrated stent-grafts. J Endovasc Ther. 2009;16(2):137-46.

37. Nordon IM, Hinchliffe RJ, Holt PJ, et al. Modern treatment of juxtarenal abdominal aortic aneurysms with fenestrated endografting and open repair—a systematic review. Eur J Vasc Endovasc Surg 2009;38(1):35-41.

38. Technology OH. Fenestrated Endovascular Grafts for the Repair of Juxtarenal Aortic Aneurysms 2009.

39. Bakoyiannis CN, Economopoulos KP, Georgopoulos S, et al. Fenestrated and branched endografts for the treatment of thoracoabdominal aortic aneurysms: a systematic review. J Endovasc Ther 2010;17(2):201-9.

40. Nordon IM, Hinchliffe RJ, Manning B, et al. Toward an "off-the-shelf" fenestrated endograft for management of short-necked abdominal aortic aneurysms: an analysis of current graft morphological diversity. J Endovasc Ther 2010;17(1):78-85.

SECTION SIX

SURGICAL ONCOLOGY

CHAPTER FOURTEEN

Management of Retroperitoneal Sarcoma

Misra S, Chaturvedi A

INTRODUCTION

Retroperitoneal sarcomas (RPS) are uncommon neoplasms occurring in the retroperitoneum and account for 10 to 15% of all sarcomas. They have an annual incidence of 2.7 cases per million. In the UK, there are probably fewer than 250 new cases of RPS each year.[1] Nearly, 80 per cent of the neoplasms that arise in the retroperitoneum are malignant and RPS constitute nearly half of these. RPS present special therapeutic challenges because of their location and frequent intimate association with several structures in the retroperitoneum.

Despite the advancement in pathology and medical treatment for sarcomas complete surgical removal with negative margins remains the mainstay of treatment. Paediatric RPS are different from adult RPS and have a different approach to treatment. The present discussion is restricted to adult RPS. Gastrointestinal stromal tumours are not classified as RPS and hence are not discussed here.

DIAGNOSIS

Clinical Presentation

Retroperitoneal sarcomas can occur over a broad age range, but have a peak incidence in the fifth and sixth decade of life.[2] Both sexes are equally affected. RPS produce few symptoms until they are large enough to compress or invade surrounding structures. Patients usually present with a non-tender palpable mass (80–90%). They may give a history of increasing abdominal girth and vague poorly localised discomfort or pain due to stretching of peritoneum in 40 to 70% patients owing to their anatomic location in the retroperitoneum.

The other symptoms are from the mass effect of the tumour on surrounding nerves, vessels and organs.

Gastrointestinal compressive symptoms occur in 20 per cent of patients and include abdominal discomfort, nausea, emesis, early satiety, changes in bowel pattern and constipation. Rarely gastrointestinal bleeding may occur due to either invasion of a hollow viscous organ or venous congestion from vascular compression.

One-third of patients (5–27%) may have some distal neurologic sign or symptom (lower extremity neuralgia, hypoaesthesia, paraesthesia and weakness) due to impingement and invasion of lumbar and pelvic nerve plexus. Genitourinary symptoms are seen in less than 10% and include urgency, frequency, haematuria and flank pain due to ureteral obstruction with associated hydronephrosis and hydroureter.

Patients may also present with generalised symptoms such as weight loss, fatigue, anorexia and fever. Weight loss can be seen in nearly 20 per cent of patients. The aetiology of weight loss in unknown and is likely to result from tumour related hyper-metabolism, early satiety, emesis and nausea from gastrointestinal obstruction. Patient with large RPS especially liposarcomas may have weight gain despite diet changes and exercise.

High grade and rapidly expanding RPS may contain region of necrosis and patients may have constant low grade fever. Rarely patients may present with paraneoplastic syndrome of hypoglycaemia due to production of insulin like substances by large poorly differentiated liposarcomas. RPS may also be diagnosed incidentally on abdominal imaging done for other reasons.

The mean duration of symptoms ranges from 5 to 10 months before diagnosis. In 70 per cent of the patients tumours are more than 10 cm in diameter at the time of presentation. Nearly 10 to 20% of patients of RPS have metastatic disease. The most common sites for haematogenous spread are the lungs and the liver. Regional lymph node metastasis is uncommon (<5%).

General examination should include a search for café-au-lait patches and other malignancies including breast, thyroid and prostate. We should look for evidence of systemic dissemination, especially to lungs and liver.

The differential diagnosis of a retroperitoneal tumour includes lymphoma, germ cell tumour, undifferentiated carcinoma, functioning and non-functioning adrenal tumours, pancreatic tumours, and advanced gastrointestinal carcinoma. A detailed history and physical examination can help distinguish many of these entities. History of fever with night sweats (B symptoms) and nodal enlargement indicate lymphoma. In men, testicular enlargement, elevated alpha-fetoprotein and beta-human chorionic gonadotropin indicates a germ cell tumour.

Pathology

The World Health Organisation has defined 50 tumour subtypes of soft tissue sarcomas.[3] These have been classified according to the predominant type of cellular differentiation such as fat (liposarcoma), blood vessels (angiosarcoma) or fibrous tissue (fibrosarcoma) or skeletal muscle (rhabdomyosarcoma). There is no evidence to support the concept of a primitive mesenchymal stem cell being the precursor of these tumours. It is more likely that switching on a given set of genes that programme mesenchymal differentiation in any type of mesenchymal cell may give rise to any mesenchymal neoplasm.[3] Evidence from micro-array and gene chip data suggests that many histologic types of sarcomas of soft tissues (STS) have characteristic patterns of gene expression associated with the process of neoplasia and may also allow further sub-classification or prognostication or assist in the identification of therapeutic targets.[4-6]

All histologic subtypes of STS occur in the retroperitoneum. Immunohistochemistry, electron microscopy and cytogenetics may help in identifying the histologic type and subtyping RPS. The predominant sarcoma types observed in the retroperitoneum are liposarcomas (25–60%), leiomyosarcoma (12–39%), malignant fibrous histocytoma (7–21%), fibrosarcoma (4–13%) and nerve sheath tumours (3–13%).[7]

There are five histologic subtypes of liposarcomas (well differentiated, dedifferentiated, myxoid, round cell and pleomorphic) having distinctly different biological behaviour.[3] The most commonly encountered subtypes in the retroperitoneum are well differentiated liposarcoma (WDLPS) and dedifferentiated liposarcomas (DDLPS). WDLPS are indolent tumours affecting people between ages of 40 to 60 years and rarely metastasise. About a quarter of WDLPS may transform into high grade or DDLPS. DDLPS have a fast growth rate and have a tendency to metastasise, and have a worse prognosis.

For RPS, histologic grading as used for other sarcomas is followed. Grade is an important prognostic factor and the TNM staging classification clearly reflects this.[8] Several grading systems have been reported using 3 or 4 grades; however, the TNM staging system utilises a two-grade classification.

Histologic grading is based on tumour histologic type/subtype, mitoses per high power field, presence of necrosis, cellular and nuclear morphology, and degree of cellularity. The histologic grade reflects metastatic potential better than cellular classification.[9] Pathologists with expertise in sarcomas having access to optimal cytogenetic and molecular diagnostic techniques may be needed to identify and grade sarcomas. Approximately half of RPS are reported to be of high grade. Patients with high grade RPS have a median survival of 33 months compared with 149 months for low grade RPS.[10]

INVESTIGATIONS

Imaging

Imaging studies for RPS involve evaluation of the primary lesion and potential sites of metastasis. Contrast enhanced computed tomography (CT) of the abdomen and pelvis is the most useful investigation in evaluation of RPS. The use of oral and intravenous contrast is necessary to allow adequate visualisation of the surrounding vascular structures, visceral organs and skeletal structures for the assessment of resectability.[11,12] Additionally, CT accurately depicts both the heterogeneous composition and the necrotic regions of these tumours, which can aid in identification of tumour histology.[13-15]

A focal nodular/water density area within a retroperitoneal liposarcoma is suggestive of DDLPS.[15] Calcification or ossification within a liposarcoma often indicates DDLPS. CT imaging also provides information about the functional status of kidneys which is invaluable if unilateral nephrectomy is required. CT also provides adequate evaluation of liver and peritoneum for metastatic disease.

Magnetic resonance imaging (MRI) is extremely accurate at imaging RPS, but given the difficulty of obtaining high quality MRI without motion artefacts, most surgeons rely on CT. Large studies comparing CT and MRI for RPS are lacking and no study has shown a benefit of using MRI over CT for RPS.[14] MRI is a useful alternative in patients with RPS who are unable to tolerate intravenous contrast for CT. It is also indicated, if CT does not provide sufficient information regarding tumour organ involvement. T1 weighted MRI image provides improved tumour delineation and aids in preoperative planning.[14] MRI/Magnetic resonance angiography (MRA) can be useful when compromise or involvement of the aorta, vena cava or iliac vessels are suspected, but there is no standard role for MRA.[12]

Positron emission tomography (PET) uses fluorine-18-fluorodeoxyglucose (FDG) to measure tumour glucose uptake as a marker of tumour activity and can be used to quantify tumour activity as opposed to anatomic detail offered by CT and MRI. Several investigators have found that FDG uptake correlates with tumour grade, mitotic rate, cellularity and survival.[16] It has also been used to assess response to neoadjuvant chemotherapy.[17] STS may show a static tumour response or a very slow reduction in size, while PET may detect this response earlier. Newer therapies directed at specific molecular targets may be cytostatic and result in tumour growth arrest, which may indicate effective therapy for a patient as opposed to direct cell killing mechanisms and tumour shrinkage.[16] Imaging by PET would be especially useful in these situations. Currently, as in many other cancers, there is no standard role for PET in screening, diagnosis or staging of STS.

Chest CT is indicated for ruling out lung metastases and is usually performed simultaneously with the abdomen CT. Isotope bone scan is not routinely indicated. If an en bloc nephrectomy seems necessary for complete resection, adequate function of the contralateral kidney must be confirmed by contrast enhanced CT, intravenous pyelography or renal scintigraphy.

Biopsy

A preoperative biopsy is not usually indicated in patients with a resectable RPS. One should proceed to appropriate treatment without a confirmatory tissue diagnosis. A biopsy is necessary only when the diagnosis may change the preoperative therapy.[18] It is indicated when the diagnosis is in doubt, as treatments for lymphoma, germ cell tumours and RPS differ substantially. It is also indicated in patients who are being considered for preoperative radiotherapy (RT) and/or chemotherapy, patients who have unresectable tumours and patients with distant metastasis.[19]

For biopsy CT guided core needle biopsy by a posterior approach is the preferred diagnostic approach. It has been found to be safe and effective in making a diagnosis of RPS. Biopsy is obtained from solid areas in the RPS. It is usually possible to provide the histologic subtype and grade on the core biopsy specimen, but requires an experienced pathologist.

Fine needle aspiration cytology (FNAC) is usually not used for the primary diagnosis. The limitations of FNAC are small material yield, difficulty in grading of STS and its dependence on the experience, and skills of the cytopathologist. An open biopsy is usually not indicated as it is potentially dangerous, may lead to contamination of the peritoneal cavity and may delay treatment. An open biopsy is reserved for the few cases in which despite a second CT guided core biopsy diagnosis cannot be made.[14]

Staging

The International Union Against Cancer (UICC) and American Joint Committee on Cancer (AJCC) staging system (UICC/AJCC) is currently followed for RPS.[8] It is based on the histologic grade, tumour size and depth, and the presence of distant or nodal metastasis. Histologic grade, depth and tumour size are the primary determinants of UICC/AJCC staging. The UICC/AJCC staging system applies rather poorly to RPS as most tumours are more than 5 cm and all are 'deep' tumours by definition, low or high histological grade is the sole determining factor between stage I disease and stage III disease. To include other prognostic factors and correct this inconsistency a post-surgical staging system has been suggested which includes grade, completeness of resection and presence of metastasis (Table 14.1).[19,20] This risk stratification system appears to be reproducible and predicts survival more accurately. A histology based RPS staging system has also been proposed which is applicable for both primary and recurrent RPS.[21]

TABLE 14.1

The Dutch/Memorial Sloan-Kettering Cancer Centre Classification System[20]

Classification	Definition
Stage I	Low grade, complete resection, no metastases
Stage II	High grade, complete resection, no metastases
Stage III	Any grade, incomplete resection, no metastases
Stage IV	Any grade, any resection, distant metastases

MANAGEMENT

Surgery remains the principal therapeutic modality in RPS. Multimodality therapy is increasingly being investigated for RPS.[22] Due to the rarity of RPS, there is a lack of prospective randomised trials of multi-modality treatment. As a result, the optimum combination and use of radiation, and chemotherapy for RPS remains debatable.

Surgery

Surgical resection is the most important aspect of treatment of RPS and therefore, the quality of surgery is critical. RPS tend to expand and infiltrate tissue planes producing a pseudo-capsule composed of normal host tissue interfaced with fimbriae of tumour. The principles of management include complete excision (monobloc) with adequate (negative) margin of normal tissue and dissection outside the pseudo-capsule.

The primary oncologic goal is complete surgical excision with microscopic negative margins. Their large size and anatomical location limits the possibility of wide resection margins. It is also often difficult to assess the microscopic margins of the resected RPS due to their large size, large surface area and lack of definite anatomical boundaries in the retroperitoneum.

Microscopic negative resections are much less frequent in RPS compared to extremity STS. However, there are reports that show the presence of microscopic tumour positive margin of resection, is associated with an increased risk of death compared with a clean microscopic margin.[23,24] The definition of radical or compartmental resection cannot be applied to RPS. Most of the surgical excisions for RPS are considered marginal.

Complete surgical resection for RPS is defined as complete gross resection with macroscopically negative margins.[10,18-20,22,24-28] Complete tumour resection rates for RPS are between 43 to 78 per cent.[2,29,30] Few series have described very high resectability rates of over 80 per cent.[10,27,31,32] Karakousis, et al.[31] have reported resectability rates of 95 per cent and have attributed this to proper positioning, proper incisions for adequate exposure, flexibility of mind, a continuous adjustment of surgical plan according to operative findings and following the path of least resistance. This increases the safety of dissection and resectability of RPS.[31]

Midline incisions are used for resecting RPS. Several other incisions depending on the site of RPS have been described to increase the resectibility rate:

- Thoraco-abdominal incision with patient in lateral position for upper quadrant tumours
- Midline incision for midline sarcomas of the upper or mid-abdomen
- Midline incision with lateral incision into the flank in form of T for flank sarcomas
- Lower midline incision with bilateral transverse extensions from the lower end of the midline incision at the pubic symphysis for pelvic midline extension of tumour
- The abdominoinguinal incision for sarcomas of the iliac fossa, wall of the lower pelvis and those extending to the pubic bone.[31]

En bloc resection of surrounding visceral organs and adjacent structures is frequently required to obtain sufficient margin on the tumour. Rates of resection of visceral organs at the time of resection of RPS vary from 34–75 per cent.[10,27] The kidney and adrenal glands (46%) are the most commonly resected organs followed by the colon (24%), pancreas (15%) and spleen (10%).[27] The adjacent viscera or structure is resected due to tumour abutment or involvement or to improve exposure and facilitate resection of tumour. The kidneys are rarely invaded; it is the encompassment of the kidney and the involvement of hilar renal vasculature that makes the resection of the kidney often necessary. Some organs such as kidney, colon and psoas can be safely removed with very limited morbidity, others such as the spleen, the left pancreas and the diaphragm that may be juxtaposed to the tumour can be resected without adding substantial morbidity. However, some other structures (e.g. duodenum/head of the pancreas, large blood vessels and spine) cannot be resected without adding real morbidity or even risk to life. Here, the concept of 'limited marginality', i.e. a planned positive margin over a critical structure and negative margin for the rest is usually practiced. No study has documented that en bloc organ resection is an independent negative prognostic factor; however, the ability to resect a RPS significantly diminishes as the number of organs involved increases.[14]

Surgical Outcome

Local control rates for RPS range from 41 to 50% at 5 years and 18 to 40% at 10 years. The overall survival rates range from 36 to 63% at 5 years and 14 to 50% at 10 years.[22]

Some authors have advocated the need for more aggressive resection in order to obtain widest possible margin to improve local control.[33-35] They advocate en bloc resection of surrounding tissues/organs in regions located within 1 to 2 cm from the tumour. The results of such resections have nearly a 70 per cent local control at 5 years but there is no formal consensus on this approach.

RPS are considered unresectable/inoperable, if there is extensive vascular involvement (aorta, vena cava and/or iliac vessels), peritoneal implants, distant metastasis, extensive disease, involvement of the root of mesentery and involvement of spinal cord.[1,36]

Major vascular involvement has traditionally been considered a criterion for unresectability for RPS.[1,36] However, major arterial and venous resection and reconstruction has been reported with favourable results.[37,38] By this complete tumour resection was possible in 60 per cent with margin-negative resection in 40 per cent of patients and a local control rate of 82 per cent with 5-year survival rate of 66.7 per cent.[37] This aggressive surgical approach is justified in selected cases and has acceptable morbidity and mortality. However, it needs an experienced surgeon.

Palliative resection (macroscopically incomplete resections/debulking) during which gross tumour may intentionally be left in the patient does not offer any survival advantage compared to patients who undergo biopsy alone.[10,30,36] The only exception to the above recommendations regarding debulking procedures applies to retroperitoneal liposarcoma, particularly WDLPS. In these patients, debulking procedures may help in palliating symptoms and prolonging survival, as the likelihood of these tumours metastasising is minimal.[39,40]

Patients with unresectable disease may need surgery for palliation of bowel obstruction, pain or bleeding. The morbidity and mortality of the palliative procedures must be carefully weighed against the quality and duration of symptom relief.

Radiation Therapy

The high local recurrence rates of RPS after complete surgical excision has led to the investigation and use of adjuvant radiation therapy (RT) as a part of multimodality treatment of these tumours.

There is ample evidence that adjuvant RT reduces the likelihood of local recurrence for extremity sarcomas. However, the evidence supporting the use of adjuvant RT for RPS is less convincing.

Radiotherapy to the retroperitoneum is challenging because of the large field size and the presence of important sensitive visceral structures like the kidney, liver, bowel and spinal cord, which are susceptible to radiation toxicity. Radiation can be administered preoperatively, postoperatively or intra-operatively (IORT). It can be given as external-beam radiation therapy (EBRT) or brachytherapy (BT).

Due to rarity of these tumours there are only a few small prospective trials in RPS. The treatment recommendations are mostly based on consensus guidelines, few prospective trials and several retrospective studies.[4] There is no trial comparing preoperative RT with postoperative RT for RPS. Thus, there remains controversy about timing of RT. Preoperative RT is usually preferred for several reasons: Gross tumour volume is more clearly demarcated for accurate treatment planning, radiosensitive viscera are displaced by tumour outside the treatment field, biologically effective radiation dose is lower in the preoperative setting, higher radiation dose can be delivered to the tumour field because of fewer surgical adhesions, tumour is treated *in situ* prior to potential contamination of the abdomen during surgery and tumour bed is better oxygenated.[22]

Postoperative RT for RPS has several disadvantages as post-resection normal tissues move into and become adherent to the tumour bed and may receive higher radiation dose and thus have higher treatment related toxicities. The standard therapeutic postoperative dose for extremity sarcomas is 60 to 70 Gy. However, it is not possible to deliver this dose for RPS due to small bowel toxicity at doses greater than 45 Gy. Larger tumour volume is also needed for postoperative RT. Postoperative RT however, has the advantage that it allows selection of patients at highest risk of recurrence based on margin status.

IORT is usually used in combination with preoperative or postoperative RT. It delivers a single large radiation fraction (10–20 Gy) to the retroperitoneum after positioning adjacent sensitive viscera out of the treatment field and targeting the specific region or regions of the operative field believed to be at the highest risk of harbouring residual microscopic disease.[22,29,41] This boost can also be delivered by brachytherapy.[41,42] Addition of IORT and BT has shown an improvement in local control, but also a high toxicity rate of neuropathy, ureteral obstruction, hydronephrosis and small bowel obstruction.[7,41]

The use of RT (preoperative or postoperative) in addition to surgery has achieved 5-year local control rates of 51 to 71 per cent in several series.[28,42-44] Pawlik, et al.[42] reported a 95 per cent resection rate and a 5-year local recurrence free and overall survival rates of 60 per cent and 61 per cent respectively from two pro-spective studies of preoperative

RT for intermediate and high grade sarcomas. These results were favourable compared to the historical data. A 55 per cent local recurrence free survival was reported with postoperative RT compared to surgery alone in a retrospective study.[28] In a prospective study comparing preoperative RT with postoperative RT for RPS no significant difference in local control rate and survival was demonstrated, but postoperative RT was associated with a significantly higher complication rate.[43]

Chemoradiation has also been studied in the treatment of RPS mostly in phase I trials. It has been demonstrated that preoperative chemoradiation is feasible but further phase II trials are needed to clarify response rates and toxicity profile.[22]

Recently, preoperative intensity modulated radiation therapy (IMRT) has offered a new method of delivering RT for RPS. It offers higher tumour killing effects while controlling toxicity by limiting dosing to surrounding organs.[29,41,45,46] IMRT delivers 45 Gy to the planned target volume, which includes the gross tumour volume plus 1 to 1.5 cm margin. This has a smaller margin than has been historically used postoperatively. Simultaneously, integrated boost doses of 57.5 to 65 Gy at 2.3 to 2.5 Gy per fraction are delivered to the margins at risk for local recurrence.[46] With IMRT the toxicity of RT is minimal.

In summary, since local recurrence is the dominant pattern of treatment failure and tumour related death, adjuvant RT is often offered to patients and remains the only adjuvant modality which decreases local recurrences in RPS. RT is especially indicated for all intermediate and high grade RPS, patients with microscopic positive margin or inpatients in whom a margin-positive resection is anticipated. However, there remains no definitive protocol for RT delivery for RPS. Based on trends seen among recent studies, preoperative EBRT 45 to 50 Gy seems to be preferred over postoperative EBRT. The methods of boost dosing are still being investigated because of their theoretical advantage of improved targeted local control without increasing the toxicity. Currently, IMRT appears to be most promising.

Chemotherapy

Chemotherapy for RPS has been used in the neoadjuvant, adjuvant and palliative settings.

Neoadjuvant Chemotherapy

There is no consensus on use of neoadjuvant chemotherapy for RPS. Neoadjuvant chemotherapy has been used with aim to decrease the tumour size and facilitate subsequent margin negative resection. Studies, most of them non-randomised, have not shown any consistent benefit with neoadjuvant chemotherapy for RPS in down staging the disease. Its use outside a clinical trial is not indicated.[11]

Adjuvant Chemotherapy

Adjuvant chemotherapy has also been used as a means of improving distant control and survival with resectable RPS. Data relating to the efficacy of chemotherapy in the treatment of RPS have been extrapolated from studies of patients with sarcomas of various sites, including the extremity, chest and abdominal wall. A systematic meta-analysis evaluated the effect of adjuvant chemotherapy on localised resectable sarcoma in 1,953 patients from 18 trials. The outcome of local, distant and overall recurrence free survival rates were significantly better in patients who received adjuvant chemotherapy than in control group. The absolute survival benefit for the entire cohort of patients was only 4% and doxorubicin combined with ifosfamide had a statistically significant overall survival in favour of chemotherapy (P=0.01).[47]

Certain histological subtype like synovial sarcoma and myxoid liposarocma are more chemosensitive and have better response. Adjuvant chemotherapy in them needs to be evaluated further. Use of adjuvant chemotherapy for RPS is not defined outside a clinical trial.

Palliative Chemotherapy

Palliative chemotherapy for RPS is used for unresectable and metastatic disease for palliation of symptoms and control of disease progression. Doxorubicin, ifosfamide and dacarbazine (DTIC) are the most active chemotherapy agents in STS. The most commonly used regimens are MAID (Mesna, Doxorubicin, Ifosfamide, Dacarbazine) and AIM (Doxorubicin, Ifosfamide, Mesna) or single agent chemotherapy commencing with doxorubicin and then proceeding to ifosfamide, and dacarbazine. Combination chemotherapy has higher response rates and also higher toxicities compared to single agent chemotherapy. Chemotherapy has been shown to be especially beneficial for certain histopathological subtype of STS like synovial sarcoma and myxoid liposarcoma. Docetaxel and gemcitabine have been shown to be effective for leiomyosarcoma.[29]

Locally Recurrent Tumours

Local recurrence is common for RPS and nearly 50 to 60% recur locally despite complete tumour resection. High grade RPS have a higher incidence of recurrence even if resected with R0 margin. Distant metastasis is less common and is usually seen with high grade tumours. For lesions that are deemed resectable and not accompanied by distant spread surgery is the preferred treatment modality at the time of local recurrence. This is often the case in low grade RPS (mainly liposarcoma). Leiomyosarcomas, pleomorphic sarcoma or malignant peripheral nerve sheath tumour have a more aggressive systemic course in comparison to liposarcoma. They usually develop distant metastasis alone or in association with local recurrence. The likelihood of obtaining a margin-negative resection is significantly lower (57%) at the time of local recurrence and decreases with subsequent recurrences compared to complete resection of primary RPS (80%).[10] A significant number of patients experience prolonged disease free survival when all grossly evident recurrent disease can be resected.

If adjuvant therapy was not delivered at the time of initial resection, it may be considered in recurrent disease. In unresectable local recurrence the treatment is palliative.

Unresectable and Metastatic Disease

Management of unresectable RPS depends on the patients overall functional status, extent of disease and symptoms. Neoadjuvant chemotherapy with an attempt to render disease resectable can be attempted, but usually it does not produce sufficient reduction to allow surgical removal. The treatment is, therefore, palliative. Palliative options include supportive care, surgical therapy (discussed earlier), radiotherapy and chemotherapy.

In patients presenting with metastases, it is important to distinguish between widely disseminated metastases and limited metastases confined to a single organ. For patients presenting with disseminated disease the treatment is palliative. Usually, these patients receive palliative chemotherapy.

In contrast patients who present with limited metastatic disease confined to a single organ and limited tumour bulk are treated with a combination of chemotherapy, surgery and radiotherapy. The treatment of metastatic pulmonary disease in patients with RPS is extrapolated from experience in treatment of extremity sarcomas and studies that include sarcomas at all sites. Selected patients with limited pulmonary metastasis undergoing resection of metastatic disease have been shown to have a survival of 22 to 36% at 5-year.[18] Resection of hepatic metastasis has also been evaluated. Survival rates following hepatic resection have generally been less than those observed for resection of pulmonary metastatic disease.[18]

PROGNOSTIC FACTORS

RPS have a much worse prognosis than extremity STS (5-year survival rate approximately 30% vs. 65%).[1] Grade and complete tumour resection are important prognostic factors in RPS.[1] Tumour size has not been identified as a predictor of survival as most RPS are more than 5 cm at presentation. A few studies have found that certain histological subtypes (leiomyosarcoma, malignant peripheral nerve sheath tumour) are a poor prognostic factor.[22]

FUTURE DIRECTIONS

Better understanding of the underlying biology of each histological subtype will help develop newer treatment approaches that will act on specific targets involved in tumourogenesis.[6] Recently, trabectedin has shown activity in synovial sarcoma, myxoid liposarcoma and leiomyosarcoma, and is being studied to define its role in combination with other agents.[29] Studies have recently reported the use of targeted therapies e.g. anti-angiogenic agents, tyrosine kinase inhibitors and mammalian target of rapamycin (MTOR) inhibitors.[48] MDM2 and CDK4 antagonists targeting specific molecular defects are being investigated for WDLPS and DDLPS. Long-term benefits of more aggressive loco-regional approaches will probably be established. With the development of IMRT, RT will be more routinely incorporated into treatment. Multi-institutional trials are needed to define the role of multi-modality therapy in RPS.

Key Points for Clinical Practice

- Most RPS present with a gradually increasing abdominal mass with few initial symptoms
- Contrast enhanced CT is useful in evaluating RPS. When contrast enhanced CT is not possible MRI may be done
- A preoperative biopsy is not indicated in resectable RPS. If neoadjuvant treatment is being planned a core needle biopsy should be done
- Complete surgical excision of all disease remains the standard of care for RPS. This may involve en bloc removal of adjacent structures
- Debulking procedure for RPS does not offer any survival advantage compared to biopsy alone except in selected patients with WDLPS
- Despite complete surgical excision RPS have a high local recurrence
- RT is the only adjuvant treatment that can improve local control. Due to lack of randomised trials there is no consensus on the standard use of RT with surgery
- Preoperative RT has better tolerance than postoperative RT
- Chemotherapy currently has little role in adjuvant setting for most RPS
- Complete surgical excision of recurrent RPS improves survival
- Patients with unresectable and metastatic disease are offered palliative treatment.

REFERENCES

1. Thomas JM. Retroperitoneal sarcoma. Br J Surg. 2007;94:1057-8.
2. Storm FK, Mahvi DM. Diagnosis and management of retroperitoneal soft-tissue sarcoma. Ann Surg. 1991;214(1):2-10.

3. International Agency for Research on Cancer (IARC). Pathology and genetics of tumours of soft tissue and bone. In: Fletcher CDM, Unni KK, Mertens F (Eds). World Health Organization classification of tumours Vol. 5, Lyon: IARC Press; 2002.

4. Hueman MT, Herman JM, Ahuja N. Management of retroperitoneal sarcomas. Surg Clin North Am. 2008;88(3):583-97.

5. Singer S, Socci ND, Ambrosini G, et al. Gene expression profiling of liposarcoma identifies distinct biological types/subtypes and potential therapeutic targets in well-differentiated and dedifferentiated liposarcoma. Cancer Res. 2007;67(14):6626-36.

6. Nielsen TO, West RB. Translating gene expression into clinical care: sarcomas as a paradigm. J Clin Oncol. 2010;28(10):1796-805.

7. Liles JS, Tzeng CW, Short JJ, et al. Retroperitoneal and intra-abdominal sarcoma. Curr Probl Surg. 2009;46(6):445-503.

8. International Union Against Cancer (UICC): Tumours of bone and soft tissues: soft tissues. In: Sobin LH, Gospodarowicz MK, Wittekind C (Eds). TNM Classification of Malignant Tumors, 7th edition. New York: Wiley-Liss 2009; 151-61.

9. Coindre JM. Grading of soft tissue sarcomas: review and update. Arch Pathol Lab Med. 2006;130(10):1448-53.

10. Lewis JJ, Leung D, Woodruff JM, et al. Retroperitoneal soft-tissue sarcoma: analysis of 500 patients treated and followed at a single institution. Ann Surg. 1998;228(3):355-65.

11. Katz MH, Choi EA, Pollock RE. Current concepts in multimodality therapy for retroperitoneal sarcoma. Expert Rev Anticancer Ther. 2007;7(2):159-68.

12. Tzeng CW, Smith JK, Heslin MJ. Soft tissue sarcoma: preoperative and postoperative imaging for staging. Surg Oncol Clin N Am. 2007;16(2):389-402.

13. Francis IR, Cohan RH, Varma DG, et al. Retroperitoneal sarcomas. Cancer Imaging. 2005;5(1):89-94.

14. Feig BW. Retroperitoneal sarcomas. Surg Oncol Clin N Am. 2003;12:369-77.

15. Lahat G, Madewell JE, Anaya DA, et al. Computed tomography scan-driven selection of treatment for retroperitoneal liposarcoma histologic subtypes. Cancer. 2009;115(5):1081-90.

16. Eary JF, Conrad EU. PET imaging: update on sarcomas. Oncology (Williston Park). 2007;21(2):249-52.

17. Benz MR, Czernin J, Allen-Auerbach MS, et al. FDG-PET/CT imaging predicts histopathologic treatment responses after the initial cycle of neoadjuvant chemotherapy in high-grade soft-tissue sarcomas. Clin Cancer Res. 2009;15(8):2856-63.

18. Windham TC, Pisters PW. Retroperitoneal sarcomas. Cancer Control. 2005;12(1):36-43.

19. Mendenhall WM, Zlotecki RA, Hochwald SN, et al. Retroperitoneal soft tissue sarcoma. Cancer. 2005;104(4):669-75.

20. van Dalen T, Hennipman A, van Coevorden F, et al. Evaluation of a clinically applicable post-surgical classification system for primary retroperitoneal soft-tissue sarcoma. Ann Surg Oncol. 2004;11(5):483-90.

21. Anaya DA, Lahat G, Wang X, et al. Establishing prognosis in retroperitoneal sarcoma: a new histology-based paradigm. Ann Surg Oncol 2009;16(3):667-75.

22. Raut CP, Pisters PW. Retroperitoneal sarcomas: combined-modality treatment approaches. J Surg Oncol. 2006;94(1):81-7.

23. Erzen D, Sencar M, Novak J. Retroperitoneal sarcoma: 25 years of experience with aggressive surgical treatment at the Institute of Oncology, Ljubljana. J Surg Oncol. 2005;91(1):1-9.

24. Anaya DA, Lev DC, Pollock RE. The role of surgical margin status in retroperitoneal sarcoma. J Surg Oncol. 2008;98(8):607-10.

25. Hassan I, Park SZ, Donohue JH, et al. Operative management of primary retroperitoneal sarcomas: a reappraisal of an institutional experience. Ann Surg. 2004;239(2):244-50.

26. Ballo MT, Zagars GK, Pollock RE, et al. Retroperitoneal soft tissue sarcoma: an analysis of radiation and surgical treatment. Int J Radiat Oncol Biol Phys. 2007;67:158-63.

27. Gronchi A, Casali PG, Fiore M, et al. Retroperitoneal soft tissue sarcomas: patterns of recurrence in 167 patients treated at a single institution. Cancer. 2004;100(11):2448-55.

28. Stoeckle E, Coindre JM, Bonvalot S, et al. Prognostic factors in retroperitoneal sarcoma: a multivariate analysis of a series of 165 patients of the French Cancer Center Federation Sarcoma Group. Cancer. 2001;92(2):359-68.

29. Thomas DM, O'Sullivan B, Gronchi A. Current concepts and future perspectives in retroperitoneal soft-tissue sarcoma management. Expert Rev Anticancer Ther. 2009;9(8):1145-57.

30. Kilkenny JW 3rd, Bland KI, Copeland EM 3rd. Retroperitoneal sarcoma: the University of Florida experience. J Am Coll Surg. 1996;182(4):329-39.

31. Karakousis CP, Kontzoglou K, Driscoll DL. Resectability of retroperitoneal sarcomas: a matter of surgical technique? Eur J Surg Oncol. 1995;21(6):617-22.

32. Ferrario T, Karakousis CP. Retroperitoneal sarcomas: grade and survival. Arch Surg. 2003;138(3):248-51.

33. Gronchi A, Lo Vullo S, Fiore M, et al. Aggressive surgical policies in a retrospectively reviewed single-institution case series of retroperitoneal soft tissue sarcoma patients. J Clin Oncol. 2009;27(1):24-30.

34. Bonvalot S, Rivoire M, Castaing M, et al. Primary retroperitoneal sarcomas: a multivariate analysis of surgical factors associated with local control. J Clin Oncol. 2009;27(1):31-7.

35. Gholami S, Jacobs CD, Kapp DS, et al. The value of surgery for retroperitoneal sarcoma. Sarcoma. 2009;2009:605840.

36. Jaques DP, Coit DG, Hajdu SI, et al. Management of primary and recurrent soft-tissue sarcoma of the retroperitoneum. Ann Surg. 1990;212(1):51-9.

37. Schwarzbach MH, Hormann Y, Hinz U, et al. Clinical results of surgery for retroperitoneal sarcoma with major blood vessel involvement. J Vasc Surg 2006;44(1):46-55.

38. Fueglistaler P, Gurke L, Stierli P, et al. Major vascular resection and prosthetic replacement for retroperitoneal tumors. World J Surg. 2006;30(7):1344-9.

39. Shibata D, Lewis JJ, Leung DH, et al. Is there a role for incomplete resection in the management of retroperitoneal liposarcomas? J Am Coll Surg. 2001;193:373-9.

40. Neuhaus SJ, Barry P, Clark MA, et al. Surgical management of primary and recurrent retroperitoneal liposarcoma. Br J Surg. 2005;92(2):246-52.

41. Tzeng CW, Fiveash JB, Heslin MJ. Radiation therapy for retroperitoneal sarcoma. Expert Rev Anticancer Ther. 2006;6:1251-60.

42. Pawlik TM, Pisters PW, Mikula L, et al. Long-term results of two prospective trials of preoperative external beam radiotherapy for localized intermediate- or high-grade retroperitoneal soft tissue sarcoma. Ann Surg Oncol. 2006;13(4):508-17.

43. Zlotecki RA, Katz TS, Morris CG, et al. Adjuvant radiation therapy for resectable retroperitoneal soft tissue sarcoma: the University of Florida experience. Am J Clin Oncol. 2005;28(3):310-6.

44. Feng M, Murphy J, Griffith KA, et al. Long-term outcomes after radiotherapy for retroperitoneal and deep truncal sarcoma. Int J Radiat Oncol Biol Phys. 2007;69(1):103-10.

45. Bossi A, De Wever I, Van Limbergen E, et al. Intensity modulated radiation-therapy for preoperative posterior abdominal wall irradiation of retroperitoneal liposarcomas. Int J Radiat Oncol Biol Phys. 2007;67(1):164-70.

46. Tzeng CW, Fiveash JB, Popple RA, et al. Preoperative radiation therapy with selective dose escalation to the margin at risk for retroperitoneal sarcoma. Cancer. 2006;107(2):371-9.

47. Pervaiz N, Colterjohn N, Farrokhyar F, et al. A systematic meta-analysis of randomized controlled trials of adjuvant chemotherapy for localized resectable soft-tissue sarcoma. Cancer. 2008;113(3):573-81.

48. Tap WD, Federman N, Eilber FC. Targeted therapies for soft-tissue sarcomas. Expert Rev Anticancer Ther. 2007;7(5):725-33.

SECTION SEVEN

CLINICAL TRIALS

Randomised Clinical Trials and Meta-analyses in Surgery 2010

Franks J, Taylor I

INTRODUCTION

In recent years managing patients according to the 'gold standard' has become the cornerstone of good surgical practise. Randomised clinical trials and meta-analyses, related to surgery, provide the foundation necessary to support an evolving evidence based practise. In this chapter, a selection of 2010 publications related to surgical topics are summarised.

GENERAL

Changes in surgical practise are driven by many external factors. Patient expectation has increasingly influenced management. It is not uncommon for patients to focus on the morbidity associated with surgical procedures. Areas which are commonly explored by patients include complications associated with the wound in particular, surgical site infections as well as postoperative pain. In addition patients consider the long-term sequelae of poor cosmesis and hernias.

Technological advances have resulted in numerous options for both abdominal incision and closure. The short and long-term results of midline abdominal incisions in patients undergoing surgery for gastrointestinal malignancies were compared when made with either a scalpel or electrocautery.[1] There was no statistically significant difference in the incidence of wound infection in the early postoperative period or incisional hernia. The method of abdominal opening therefore, remains a matter of surgical preference.

The 'Jenkins rule' is commonly quoted as the technique of choice for the closure of the fascial layer of a midline laparotomy.[2] A recent publication considered the results of five systematic reviews and 14 trials including 6,752 midline incisions.[3] Analysis confirmed that there was a significantly lower hernia rate using a continuous (vs. interrupted) technique (OR:0.59; P=0.001). The results also showed that using a slowly absorbable suture (vs. rapid-absorbable) material (OR:0.65; P=0.009) was acceptable in the elective setting.

The technique used for the closure of the skin following midline laparotomy has also been compared in a prospective randomised trial. Patients undergoing open elective colectomy for benign or malignant indications were allocated to skin closure with 2-octyl cyanoacrylate (Dermabond) or skin staples.[4] No significant difference in cosmetic outcomes was seen between the two groups. However, there was a trend to improved outcome in the 2-octyl cyanoacrylate group along with higher patient satisfaction scores. 2-octyl cyanoacrylate has the practical advantage of requiring no further input, such as additional dressing, once in place. It is also waterproof allowing the patients to wash immediately after surgery. The time taken to close the wound with 2-octyl cyanoacrylate was however shown to be longer. No difference in rates of infection was demonstrated.

Key Points

- When considering a midline laparotomy, the rate of surgical site infection and incisional hernia are not altered by using either a scalpel or electrocautery to make the incision
- The fascial layer should be closed with a continuous slowly absorbable suture in the elective setting
- Skin closure with 2-octyl cyanoacrylate (Dermabond) has a high patient satisfaction score with comparable cosmesis and no increase in infection rates.

Adherence to evidence based surgical techniques will reduce but not eliminate sequelae such as wound breakdown. Vacuum dressings are now established as a method used to treat this complication. There can be a delay in initiating this management owing to the availability of the machines specifically designed for this purpose. In addition, the equipment is expensive and requires adequate training to be used correctly. A recently published randomised clinical trial has compared conventional saline soaked gauze dressings with a home-made wound vacuum dressing system (HM-VAC) assembled from tools available in most operating room worldwide.[5] The time required to achieve complete healing was 16 days in the HM-VAC group compared to 25 days in the conventional group (P=0.013). To treat a case with HM-VAC was only $89 more expensive than gauze and saline dressings.

Key Point

- Home-made wound vacuum dressing system results in significantly faster healing of complex wounds using equipment readily available in most hospitals. The cost of this system does not prohibit its use in resource-poor hospitals.

Optimal pain control reduces postoperative complications such as basal atelectasis and subsequent chest infections, as well as being paramount to patient centered care. A systematic review of the literature has looked at the results of seven randomised clinical trials investigating the effect of the transversus abdominis plane (TAP) block on postoperative pain.[6] This is a newly described peripheral block involving the nerves of the anterior abdominal wall which has been developed for postoperative pain control after gynaecological and abdominal surgery. Most studies have demonstrated clinically significant reductions of postoperative opioid requirements and pain, as well as some effects on opioid-related side effects such as sedation and postoperative nausea and vomiting.

Appendicitis remains the most common general surgical emergency. One randomised controlled trial has looked at the effectiveness of the TAP block in children undergoing open appendicectomy.[7] Forty children were randomised to undergo unilateral TAP block, after induction of anaesthesia, with ropivacaine 75 per cent (2.5 mg/Kg) or an equal volume of saline (0.3 ml/Kg) in addition to standard postoperative analgesia. The TAP block reduced mean morphine requirements in the first 48 postoperative hours as well as visual analogue pain scores at rest and on movement. In addition there were no complications attributable to the TAP block.

Key Point

- Transversus abdominis plane (TAP) block is an effective component of a multimodal analgesic regimen.

The effect of pre-emptive analgesia on postoperative pain is firmly established. Preoperative nonsteroidal anti-inflammatory drugs (NSAIDs) have been shown to effectively reduce postoperative pain in surgical patients treated electively for non-inflammatory conditions such as inguinal hernia. Two recently published trials have looked at the impact of administering preoperative rectal indomethacin on postoperative pain after open appendicectomy[8] and cholecystectomy.[9] In both studies patients who received this NSAID preoperatively experienced significantly less postoperative pain. This was demonstrated by their visual analogue scale results. In addition they required less total opioid.

The analgesic and antiemetic properties of steroids, such as dexamethasone, are well-known leading to its routine incorporation in anaesthetic premedication. The effect of preoperative dexamethasone on postoperative symptoms in patients undergoing laparoscopic cholecystectomy has been explored by two trials. In one prospective randomised placebo controlled trial patients received intravenous placebo, 4 mg or 8 mg of dexamethasone.[10] The need for breakthrough analgesia was significantly less in the 8 mg group when compared to the placebo group (P=0.008) and 4 mg group (P=0.029). No difference in analgesic requirement was found between the 4 mg and placebo group. In a different study, patients were randomised to 8 mg of dexamethasone or placebo.[11] The patients who received dexamethasone reported less postoperative pain with significantly fewer patients experiencing postoperative nausea and vomiting up to 12 hours after surgery. The need for ondansetron in the treatment group was significantly lower than in the placebo group and less fatigue was reported.

Key Points

- Preoperative administration of rectal NSAIDs is an effective pre-emptive analgesia reducing both patients postoperative pain and opioid requirements
- Preoperatively, 8 mg of dexamethasone is effective in reducing the analgesic requirement and postoperative nausea and vomiting of patients undergoing laparoscopic cholecystectomy.

In order to improve outcome and reduce morbidity many units are using protocols to guide surgical management after major complex surgical procedures. Restrictions in working hours in Europe and reliance on full shifts with multiple handovers between doctors in a 24 hours period is likely to increase the implementation of this pattern of surgical management.

The complications associated with long-term mechanical ventilation are well known. In the last year a prospective, randomised controlled trial has compared the duration of mechanical ventilation for 100 patients who required more than 24 hours of treatment following intra-abdominal surgery.[12] Patients were assigned to receive either protocol based nurse-directed weaning or physician-directed weaning from mechanical ventilation. Patients assigned to the protocol arm of the trial underwent daily screening and a spontaneous breathing trial by the nursing staff. The median duration of mechanical ventilation was 40 and 72 hours (P<0.001) in the protocol-directed and physician directed groups respectively. Two patients were re-intubated within the first 72 hours after extubation in the protocol-directed group compared to three in the physician-directed group (p=0.61).

Key Point

- Protocol directed weaning results in a shorter duration of mechanical ventilation in patients who have undergone intra-abdominal surgery.

Invasive monitoring aims to identify inadequate tissue perfusion. It has been integrated into the standard management of patients undergoing major surgery to enable rapid and appropriate adjustments to their management. In most hospitals this takes place in a high dependency or post-anaesthetic care unit. Regimes for perioperative fluid management are increasingly seen in the protocols used to manage these complex patients. A randomised trial looked at the outcome of patients who underwent surgery for gastrointestinal malignancy and were managed with a restricted intravenous fluid regime.[13] The patients were randomised into two groups. One group received additional fluid and electrolytes according to clinical criteria. The other group had their serum lactate closely monitored and were given additional fluid to maintain this at a normal level. In the group of patients whose fluid was adjusted according to their lactate, their supplementary fluid was started within the first 12 hours more frequently than in the standard care group (74% vs. 37%). The patients who received supplementary fluid according to clinical criteria alone had significantly worse outcomes. Their overall complication rate was 85 per cent, with major complications seen in 44 per cent of patients compared to 45 per cent and 16 per cent (P=0.023 and P=0.001) respectively for the patients who had serial monitoring of their serum lactate.

Key Point

- Close monitoring of serum lactate in the perioperative and early postoperative period with adjustment of intravenous fluid may improve early detection and correction of inadequate tissue perfusion with a subsequent reduction in complications.

The scoring systems used to determine the prognosis of critically ill patients invariably assess each system, either directly or indirectly, to determine function and predict mortality. Inadequate gut function is common in critically ill surgical patients and may be associated with a poor prognosis similar to that of other single organ failures. However, it is difficult to measure and treatment options are limited. The role of gut-specific nutrients (GSNs) has been evaluated in one study to determine if they could stimulate the return of gut function in critically ill surgical patients and what effect this would have on outcomes.[14] Twenty-five patients intolerant to enteral feeding were randomised to receive GSN or placebo for one month. The patients were followed for three months. GSN was associated with a quicker return of normal gut function (median 164 vs. 214 hours, P=0.016) and a lower incidence of sepsis (4 vs. 13 patients, P=0.015). At 3 months there were fewer deaths in the treatment arm but this did not reach significance (2 vs. 7 deaths, P=0.138).

Key Point

- Gut-specific nutrients (GSNs) expedite the return of gut function in critically ill patients and improve outcomes.

LAPAROSCOPIC SURGERY

Laparoscopic surgery is now so deeply incorporated into surgery that it has established its own subspeciality. Along with all other sub-specialties developments in both technology and technique allow new procedures to be performed. The Da Vinci surgical system (DVSS) is an emerging laparoscopic technology whose use is being increasingly seen. A systematic review of 31 studies, six of them randomised controlled trials, involving 2,166 patients compared DVSS with conventional laparoscopic surgery.[15] The procedures undertaken included fundoplication, Heller myotomy, gastric bypass, gastrectomy, bariatric surgery, cholecystectomy, splenectomy, colorectal resection and rectopexy. DVSS was demonstrated to be associated with fewer Heller myotomy-related perforations, a more rapid intestinal recovery time after gastrectomy, a longer operative time for cholecystectomy but a shorter hospital stay, longer colorectal resection surgery times and a larger number of conversions to open surgery during gastric bypass. These results should however be interpreted with caution. Particular attention should be paid to future studies which include surgery performed for oncological indications and as such include outcomes such as survival.

Key Point

- Da Vinci surgical system (DVSS) is an emerging laparoscopic technology which offers certain advantages with respect to Heller myotomy, gastrectomy and cholecystectomy.

Hand assisted laparoscopic surgery (HALS) is a new addition to minimal access surgery. This technique allows surgeons to insert a hand through a small incision via a special pressurised sleeve. The main advantage is a gain in tactile sense during laparoscopic surgical procedures. As HALS gains popularity, studies are emerging to determine if this alteration to the laparoscopic technique allows it to preserve its well documented advantages over more traditional surgical approaches. One trial has compared HALS and open splenectomy in splenomegaly cases.[16] The clinical results of 27 patients prospectively randomised to either procedure have been published. The benefit of HALS over open splenectomy were a shorter abdominal incision (P=0.012), less postoperative pain (P=0.0002) and shorter hospital stay (P=0.004).

Key Point

- Hand assisted laparoscopic surgery (HALS) for splenectomy retains the advantages of laparoscopic surgery by maintaining a significantly smaller incision, less postoperative pain and shorter hospital stay whilst conferring the benefits of tactile strength and atraumatic manipulation of enlarged spleens.

Laparoscopic cholecystectomy is currently the gold standard procedure for gallstones which require surgical intervention. A standard laparoscopic cholecystectomy uses four trocars leading to an accumulative break in the continuity of the abdominal wall of 25 to 30 mm. New techniques are now being used which reduce either the size or number of the ports. There has been an increasing number of publications looking at either mini-laparoscopic cholecystectomy (MLC), which uses smaller instruments, typically the trocars are 10 mm (umbilical), 5 mm (epigastric) and 2 mm (subcostal and lateral) or single incision laparoscopic cholecystectomy (SILC). One randomised clinical trial has compared these two techniques in the treatment of symptomatic gallstones.[17] The outcome of the two groups of patients was prospectively compared. Surgical complications, postoperative pain scores, analgesic requirements and time to return to work were similar for both procedures. Statistically significant advantages of SILC were a shorter hospital stay, shorter total wound length and better cosmetic appearance. The duration of operation was significantly shorter for MLC.

Key Point

- Single incision laparoscopic cholecystectomy (SILC) and mini-laparoscopic cholecystectomy (MLC) are gaining increasing momentum in the treatment of symptomatic gallstones. SILC is superior to MLC in terms of cosmetic outcome but not in postoperative pain and requirement for analgesics.

The number of people that require kidney transplantation is increasing in all western societies. This has led to an increase in the demand for kidney transplantation. The suitability of an individual for living kidney donation depends on many factors not least on their willingness to donate. A randomised clinical trial has looked at the safety and efficacy of laparoscopic donor nephrectomy in comparison with short-incision open donor nephrectomy.[18] There was no donor death or allograft thrombosis in either group. The first warm ischaemic time and duration of operation were significantly longer for the laparoscopic group of patients. However, the laparoscopic approach led to a reduction in parenteral morphine requirement and an earlier return to employment. Postoperative respiratory function was also noted to be improved after laparoscopic nephrectomy. There were more complications per donor in the open group. At a median follow-up of 74 months there were no differences in renal function or allograft survival between the groups.

Key Point

- Laparoscopic nephrectomy is a safe procedure which removes some of the disincentives to live donation without compromising the outcome of the recipient transplant.

UPPER GASTROINTESTINAL

Gastro-oesophageal Reflux Disease

The superiority of surgery over medical management in the treatment of gastro-oesophageal reflux disease (GORD) has led to laparoscopic Nissen fundoplication (LNF) becoming the procedure of choice for the management of this condition. In the immediate postoperative period the incidence of para-oesophageal herniation is as high as 7 per cent. A prospective randomised trial has looked at the affect combining posterior gastropexy with LNF has on the postoperative results of this surgical procedure.[19] The gastropexy was performed with one stitch between the posterior wall of the wrap and the crura near the arcuate ligament. In the group of patients who were treated by both LNF and gastropexy no para-oesophageal hernias were diagnosed compared to one in the LNF only group which required re-operation. The gastropexy did not cause a significant difference in postoperative dysphagia or healing of Barrett's oesophagus on subsequent endoscopy.

Key Point

- Laparoscopic Nissen fundoplication (LNF) combined with posterior gastropexy may prevent postoperative herniation in the surgical treatment of GORD providing better early and long-term postoperative results.

Gastric Carcinoma

Surgical resection is the mainstay of treatment for operable gastric carcinoma. Despite this there is still considerable controversy in the literature with regard to the appropriateness of performing radical gastrectomy with D2 dissection, owing to the complications and high mortality associated with it. A randomised clinical trial compared the outcomes of D1 and D2 gastrectomy in specialised centres.[20] Two hundred sixty-seven patients with operable gastric cancer were randomly assigned to either a D1 or D2 procedure in five centres. In the intention to treat analysis, the overall morbidity rate after D1 and D2 resections was 12 per cent and 17.9 per cent respectively (P=0.178). There was a single duodenal stump leak in the D2 arm (0.7%). Thirty days postoperative mortality rate was 3 per cent after D1 and 2.2 per cent are D2 gastrectomy.

Key Point

- The radical treatment of gastric cancer by D2 gastrectomy is a safe option with acceptable morbidity and mortality rates when performed in specialised centres.

Enhanced recovery is being implemented across surgical specialities. Patients undergoing colorectal resections have been shown to benefit from a comprehensive programme of perioperative and postoperative care. There has been renewed interest in applying these principles to gastric surgery resulting in the publication of two randomised trials. One looked at the outcome of gastrectomy patients who had undergone optimised perioperative care compared to conventional treatment.[21] The optimised group had a significantly shorter hospital stay compared to the conventional care group (P<0.001). In addition the duration of urinary and abdominal drainage was less (P<0.001) as well as an earlier recovery of gut function (P<0.001) and lower inflammatory markers. A different trial also published this year randomised patients, with gastric cancer, into fast-track and conventional surgery groups.[22] The fast track group had no more complications with a significantly shorter duration of fever and hospital stay as well as higher quality of life scores on hospital discharge (all P<0.05).

Key Point

- Enhanced recovery in gastrectomy patients shortens hospital stay as well as speeding up the return of gut function and reducing postoperative stress reactions without increasing complications.

Despite potentially curative resection of gastric cancer between 50 to 90 per cent of patients die of disease relapse. A meta-analysis of all randomised clinical trials has been performed aiming to quantify the benefit of adjuvant chemotherapy after complete resection over surgery alone.[23] Individual patient data was available from 17 trials (3,838 patients). Adjuvant chemotherapy was associated with a statistically significant benefit in terms of overall survival (HR 0.82) and disease free survival (HR 0.82). Five-year overall survival increased from 49.6 per cent to 55.3 per cent with chemotherapy.

Gastric Outlet Obstruction

Despite improvements in the management of upper GI and pancreatic cancers palliative treatments are still required to treat malignant gastric outlet obstruction. The SUSTENT study[24] randomised patients into gastrojejunostomy and stent placement. Food intake improved more rapidly after stent placement but long-term relief of obstructive symptoms was better after gastrojejunostomy. More major complications ($P=0.02$) occurred and more re-interventions were performed ($P<0.01$) after stent placement than after gastrojejunostomy.

HEPATO-PANCREATIC AND BILIARY

Pancreatic Surgery

The emergency admission of a patient with pancreatitis is a common occurrence on a general surgical take. The majority of these admissions will not require surgery and can be managed without transfer to a specialised unit. The outcome for patients with pancreatitis is determined by its severity. Several scoring systems have proven validity, each aims to predict which cases will develop severe pancreatitis. Severe pancreatitis has many recognised sequelae, among them is pancreatic necrosis. If it becomes infected the mortality increases. In some units antibiotics are routinely given to patients with CT proven necrosis; however, the role of prophylactic antibiotics in this setting has not been established with opponents raising concerns over resistance and fungal infection.

Seven randomised controlled trials studies, including 404 patients were reviewed to determine the efficacy and safety of prophylactic antibiotics in acute pancreatitis complicated by CT proven pancreatic necrosis.[25] Overall there was no statistically significant reduction of infected pancreatic necrosis rates or mortality with therapy. Beta-lactam antibiotic prophylaxis resulted in lower mortality (9.4% treatment vs.

15% controls) and less infected pancreatic necrosis (16.8% treatment vs. 24.2% controls); however, this did not reach statistical significance. Imipenem on its own showed no difference in the incidence of mortality but there was a significant reduction in the rate of pancreatic infection (P=0.02 RR 0.34).

Key Point

- Imipenem significantly deceases the rate of infection of pancreatic necrosis; however, this does not translate to a reduction in the incidence of mortality.

Necrotising pancreatitis with necrotic tissue is associated with a high rate of complications and death. Open necrosectomy is the standard treatment. There has recently been renewed interest in adopting a minimally invasive step-up approach. This consists of percutaneous drainage followed by, if necessary, minimally invasive retroperitoneal necrosectomy. A multicentre study randomised patients into the above two treatment arms.[26] Major complications including: new-onset multiple organ failure, multiple systemic complications, perforation of a visceral organ, enterocutaneous fistula or bleeding occurred in 69 per cent of patients in the open necrosectomy arm and 40 per cent in the step-up approach arm (P=0.006). Of the patients assigned to the step-up arm 35 per cent were treated with percutaneous drainage only. New onset multiorgan failure, incisional hernia and new onset diabetes occurred statistically less in the step-up arm. The rate of death did not differ significantly between the groups.

Key Point

- A minimally invasive step-up approach for the treatment of necrotising pancreatitis and infected necrotic tissue reduces the rate of major complications.

The high morbidity and mortality of severe pancreatitis has led to the exploration of noble management strategies to improve outcome. One randomised trial has looked at the therapeutic effects of haemofiltration combined with peritoneal filtration in the treatment of severe acute pancreatitis.[27] The mean time of abdominal pain relief, amelioration of abdominal discomfort, decrease in computed tomographic scores, acute physiology and chronic health enquiry II scores, the mean length of stay and cost of hospitalisation of the treatment group were significantly shorter or less then the control group. Inflammatory cytokines including TNFα, IL-6 and IL-8 were decreased significantly in the serum and ascites of the dialysis group.

Biliary

Endoscopic retrograde cholangiopancreatography plus sphincterotomy (ERCP/S) is recognised as the standard treatment of gallstones in the common bile duct. This is conventionally followed by laparoscopic cholecystectomy. Advances in both laparoscopic techniques and training plus increased availability of specialised equipment has resulted in an increasing number of patients being managed by laparoscopic cholecystectomy plus laparoscopic common bile duct exploration. A study has compared the outcome parameters for good risk patients (ASA I and II) with classic symptoms and signs of gallstone disease plus appropriate abdominal imaging and laboratory results into two treatment arms: ERCP/S followed by laparoscopic cholecystectomy or laparoscopic cholecystectomy plus laparoscopic common bile duct exploration.[28] Efficacy of stone clearance was equivalent for both groups. However, the time from first procedure to discharge was significantly shorter for the patients managed entirely laparoscopically (P<0.001). The patient acceptance and quality of life scores were equivalent for both groups.

Choledochotomy and removal of common bile duct stones was initially described as an open technique. The convention was to close the duct with a T-tube which remained *in situ* for several weeks. As laparoscopic exploration of the biliary tree gains popularity the technique is being adapted to bring it into line with other minimal access procedures where the aim is a reduction in trauma, faster recovery and shorter hospital stay. T-tube insertion seems to counteract these benefits. A study randomised patients who underwent laparoscopic common bile duct exploration into those who had a T-tube inserted and those who underwent primary closure.[29] The group who did not have a drain inserted had a significantly shorter operative time and postoperative stay in addition the incidence of postoperative and biliary complications were statistically lower.

The overall duration of hospitalisation when managed completely laparoscopically is shorter with subsequent reduction in cost
- Laparoscopic common bile duct exploration with primary closure is feasible and as safe as T-tube insertion.

COLORECTAL

In line with all subspecialties colorectal surgery is adapting established surgical approaches in order to offer more minimal access surgery. In addition, the role of enhanced recovery has been championed by colorectal surgery. Recently, several published studies have looked at the best way to manage postoperative pain, reduce the duration of an ileus as well as improve management of postoperative complications such as adhesions.

Laparoscopically assisted surgery is a validated technique for colorectal cancer. Its role in the surgical treatment of benign conditions such as bowel endometriosis has until now not been addressed. Fifty five women with colorectal endometriosis were randomly assigned to laparoscopically assisted or open colorectal surgery.[30] Overall a significant improvement in gastrointestinal symptoms, such as diarrhoea, gynaecological symptoms, such as dysmenorrhoea and general symptoms, such as back pain, were observed. Median blood loss was lower in the laparoscopic group (P<0.05). The total number of complications was higher in the open group (P=0.04). The pregnancy rate was higher in the laparoscopic group (P=0.006) and the cumulative pregnancy rate was 60 per cent. No difference in quality of life was noted between the two groups.

Key Point

- Laparoscopy is a safe option for women with severe bowel endometriosis requiring resection. In addition, it offers a higher pregnancy rate than open surgery with improvements in symptoms and quality of life.

Postoperative epidural analgesia is recognised to be the gold standard method of managing pain in patients who undergo laparotomy. It has been shown to shorten ileus duration and hospital stay after colon surgery when compared with the use of systemic opioids. However, epidural placement is not suitable for all patients. An intravenous (IV) infusion of local anaesthetic has been shown to have a similar effect on outcome in patients undergoing colon surgery. A randomised clinical trial was conducted to directly compare these two treatments in patients who had undergone open colon surgery.[31] Twenty-two patients were randomised to IV lidocaine (1 mg/min in patients <70 Kg, 2 mg/min in patients >70 Kg) and twenty patients to epidural therapy (bupivacaine 0.125% + hydromorphine 6 µg/ml at 10 ml/hr started within an hour of the end of surgery). The median pain scores, return to bowel function and hospital length of stay showed no statistical difference between the two groups.

Key Point

- An IV infusion of local anaesthetic may be an effective alternative to epidural therapy in patients undergoing laparotomy in whom epidural anaesthesia is contraindicated or not desired.

It is not uncommon for patients who have previously undergone surgery to present as an emergency with small bowel obstruction secondary to adhesions. Gastrografin is commonly used to aid diagnosis and assess the need for surgical intervention. A trial randomised patients into control and gastrografin groups to assess the diagnostic and therapeutic effect of this practise.[32] The gastrografin group were administered 100 ml of contrast through a nasogastric tube. Obstruction was considered complete if no contrast was seen in the colon at 24 hours. Patients with gastrografin in the colon within 24 hours were considered to be partially obstructed and were submitted to non-operative treatment. The patients were operated on, if they developed signs of strangulation or failed to improve within 48 hours. The operative rate was 14.5 per cent for the gastrografin group compared to 34.5 per cent in the control group (P=0.04). The time from admission to resolution of symptoms was significantly lower in the gastrografin group, 19.5 hours compared to 42.6 hours in the control group (P=0.001), with a shorter length of stay.

Key Point

- Oral gastrografin speeds up resolution of symptoms and reduces the operation rate in patients with adhesive small bowel obstruction.

Colorectal Cancer

Colorectal cancer is the third most common cancer worldwide and has a high mortality rate. As the pathogenesis of this disease is understood with a stepwise progression from adenoma to carcinoma, it is a suitable condition for screening according to Wilson's criteria. A recently published randomised controlled trial was undertaken in 14 UK centres to determine if only one flexible screening sigmoidoscopy between 55 and 64 years of age could substantially reduce colorectal cancer incidence and mortality.[33]

1,13,195 people were assigned to the control group and 57,237 to the intervention group, of whom 1,12,939 and 57,099, respectively were included in the final analyses. 40,674 (71%) underwent flexible sigmoidoscopy. The published results are based on a median follow-up of 11.2 years. In per-protocol analyses, adjusted for self-selection bias in the intervention group, incidence of colorectal cancer in people attending screening was reduced by 33 per cent (HR 0.67) and mortality by 43 per cent (HR 0.57). Incidence of distal colorectal cancer (rectum and sigmoid colon) was reduced by 50 per cent. The numbers needed to be screened to prevent one colorectal cancer diagnosis or death, by the end of the study period, were 191 and 489, respectively.

Key Point

- Flexible sigmoidoscopy is a safe and practical test. It is a suitable screening tool and can be offered once between the ages of 55 and 64 years to confer a substantial and lasting benefit.

Fissure in Ano

Fissure in ano is one of a number of benign conditions which are frequently referred to the colorectal clinic for specialist management. A Cochrane systematic review of the operative procedures for anal fissure has been updated to determine the best technique for fissure surgery.[34] Twenty-four trials encompassing 3,475 patients are included in the review. The two endpoints used in this meta-analysis were persistence of fissure and postoperative incontinence to flatus. Anal stretch had a higher risk of fissure persistence than internal sphincterotomy. It also has a significantly higher risk of minor incontinence than sphincterotomy. The combined results of open versus closed lateral internal sphincterotomy showed little difference between the two procedures for both endpoints.

The complications of surgery for anal fissure, although rare, have an understandably negative impact on a patient's quality of life. There has therefore been renewed interest in finding an alternative treatment strategy that confers high rates of fissure healing without the risk of long-term complications. Botulinum toxin has been used successfully to fulfil this role. The technique for optimal injection has not yet been established. A recent study has compared bilateral (20 units into each side of the internal anal sphincter) versus posterior injection (25 units in the midline) of botulinum toxin.[35] The mean time to pain relief and healing did not show any significant difference between the two groups. Treatment failure and recurrence were also noted not to show any significant difference.

Key Points

- Anal stretch and posterior midline sphincterotomy should be abandoned in the treatment of chronic anal fissure
- Open and closed partial lateral sphincterotomy appear to be equally efficacious and therefore the method used is a matter of surgeons preference
- Botulinum toxin is an effective treatment for acute anal fissure. A single posterior injection is easier and less painful than bilateral injections and is as effective in pain relief and fissure healing.

HERNIA

The two most common procedures for open tension free repair of groin hernias are the Lichtenstein operation and the mesh plug technique. Out of 167 patients with inguinal hernias, 155 patient were randomised to a plug and mesh procedure with either sutures, human fibrin glue or N-butyl-2-cyanoacrylate for mesh fixation.[36] The overall morbidity rate was 38.98 per cent in the suture group, 9.62 per cent in the fibrin glue and 10.71 per cent in the N-butyl-2-cyanoacrylate. There was no significant difference between the groups in terms of mean postoperative stay and mean time to return to work. There was no recurrence in any of the groups. Two cases (3.39%) of chronic pain were reported in patients in the suture group.

Key Point

- The use of human fibrin glue or N-butyl-2-cyanoacrylate is better tolerated than sutures in patients undergoing open tension-free plug and mesh repair of groin hernias.

BREAST

The aetiology of breast cancer is a subject that is commonly touched on in both scientific journals and the health sections of the national press. A recently published study aimed to determine the effects of therapy with oestrogen and progesterone on cumulative breast cancer incidence and mortality in postmenopausal women after a mean follow-up of 11 years.[37] A total of 16,608 postmenopausal women aged 50 to 79 years with no prior hysterectomy from 40 centres were randomly assigned to receive combined equine oestrogens (0.625 mg/d) plus medroxyprogesterone acetate (2.5 mg/d) or placebo pill. In the intention-to-treat analyses the treatment arm was associated with more invasive breast cancers compared with placebo (HR 1.25). Breast cancers in the treatment group were similar in histology and grade but more likely to be node positive (HR 1.78). There were also more deaths directly attributed to breast cancer (HR 1.96) as well as more deaths from all causes occurring after breast cancer diagnosis (HR 1.57) in the treatment arm.

Key Point

- Oestrogen and progesterone are associated with greater breast cancer incidence in postmenopausal women. The breast cancers are more likely to be node positive at diagnosis
- Breast cancer mortality also appears to be increased in women who have been treated with oestrogen and progesterone.

Key Points for Clinical Practice

- The fascial layer should be closed with a continuous slowly absorbable suture in the elective setting.
- Transversus abdominis plane (TAP) block is an effective component of a multimodal analgesic regimen.
- Protocol directed weaning results in a shorter duration of mechanical ventilation in patients who have undergone intra-abdominal surgery.
- Close monitoring of serum lactate in the perioperative and early postoperative period with adjustment of intravenous fluid may improve early detection and correction of inadequate tissue perfusion with a subsequent reduction in complications.
- Da Vinci surgical system (DVSS) is an emerging laparoscopic technology which offers certain advantages with respect to Heller myotomy, gastrectomy and cholecystectomy.
- Laparoscopic Nissen fundoplication (LNF) combined with posterior gastropexy may prevent postoperative herniation in the surgical treatment of GORD providing better early and long-term postoperative results.
- Postoperative adjuvant chemotherapy based on fluorouracil regimens was associated with reduced risk of death in gastric cancer compared with surgery alone.
- Gastrojejunostomy has superior outcomes compared to stent placement in the palliative management of malignant gastric outlet obstruction
- Imipenem significantly deceases the rate of infection of pancreatic necrosis; however, this does not translate to a reduction in the incidence of mortality.
- Laparoscopic common bile duct exploration with primary closure is feasible and as safe as T-tube insertion.
- Laparoscopy is a safe option for women with severe bowel endometriosis requiring resection. In addition, it offers a higher pregnancy rate than open surgery with improvements in symptoms and quality of life.

- Oral gastrografin speeds up resolution of symptoms and reduces the operation rate in patients with adhesive small bowel obstruction.
- Flexible sigmoidoscopy is a safe and practical test. It is a suitable screening tool and can be offered once between the ages of 55 and 64 years to confer a substantial and lasting benefit.
- Anal stretch and posterior midline sphincterotomy should be abandoned in the treatment of chronic anal fissure
- Botulinum toxin is an effective treatment for acute anal fissure. A single posterior injection is easier and less painful than bilateral injections and is as effective in pain relief and fissure healing.

REFERENCES

1. Eren T, Balik E, Ziyade S, et al. Do different abdominal incision techniques play a role in wound complications in patients operated on for gastrointestinal malignancies? "Scalpel vs. electrocautery". Acta Chiruriga Belgica 2010;110(4):451-6.
2. Jenkins TP. The burst abdominal wound: A mechanical approach. Br J Surg 1976;63(11):873-6.
3. Diener M, Voss S, Jenson K, et al. Elective midline laparotomy closure: The INLINE systematic review and meta-analysis. Ann Surg 2010;251(5): 843-56.
4. Ong J, Ho K, Chew M, et al. Prospective randomized study to evaluate the use of DERMABOND ProPen (2-octyl cyanoacrylate) in the closure of abdominal wounds versus closure with skin staples in patients undergoing elective colectomy. Int J Colorectal Dis 2010;25(7):899-905.
5. Perez D, Bramkamp M, Exe C, et al. Modern wound care for the poor: A randomized clinical trial comparing the vacuum system with conventional saline-soaked gauze dressings. Am J Surg 2010;199(1):14-20.
6. Peterson P, Mathiesen O, Torup H, et al. The transversus abdominis plane block: A valuable option for postoperative analgesia? A topical review. Acta Anaesthesio Scand 2010;54(5):529-35.
7. Carney J, Finnerty O, Rauf J, et al. Ipsilateral transversus abdominis plane block provides effective analgesia after appendectomy in children: A randomized controlled trial. Anesthsia and Analgesia 2010;111(4):998-1003.
8. Jangjoo A, Bahar M, Soltani E. Effect of preoperative rectal indomethacin on postoperative pain reduction after open appendectomy. J Opioid Manag 2010;6(1):63-6.
9. Bahar M, Jangjoo A, Soltani E, et al. Effect of preoperative rectal in-domethacin on postoperative pain reduction after open cholecystectomy. J Perianesth Nurs 2010;25(1):7-10.
10. Fujii Y, Itakura M. Reduction of postoperative nausea, vomiting, and analgesic requirement with dexamthasone for patients undergoing laparoscopic cholecystectomy. Surg Endosc 2010;24(3):692-6.
11. Sanchez-Rodriguez P, Fuentes-Orozco C, Gonzalez-Ojeda A. Effect of dexamethasone on postoperative symptoms in patients undergoing elective laparoscopic cholecystectomy: A randomized clinical trial. World J Surg 2010;34(5):985-900.

12. Chaiwat O, Sarima N, Niyompanitpattana K, et al. Protocol-directed vs. Physician-directed weaning from ventilator in intra-abdominal surgical patients. J Med AssocThai 2010;93(8):930-6.

13. Wenkui Y, Ning L, Jianfeng G, et al. Restricted perioperative fluid administration adjusted by serum lactate level improved outcome after major elective surgery for gastrointestinal malignancy. Surgery 2010;147(4):542-52.

14. Gatt M , MacFie J. Randomized clinical trial of gut-specific nutrients in critically ill surgical patients. Br J Surg 2010;97(11):1629-36.

15. Maeso S, Reza M, Mayol J, et al. Efficacy of the Da Vinci surgical system in abdominal surgery compared with that of laparoscopy: A systematic review and meta-analysis. Ann Surg 2010;252(2):254-62.

16. Barbaros U, Dinccag A, Sumer A, et al. Prospective randomized comparison of clinical results between hand-assisted laparoscopic and open splenectomies. Surg Endosc 2010;24(1):25-32.

17. Lee P, Lo C, Lai P, et al. Randomized clinical trial of single-incision laparoscopic cholecystectomy versus minilaparoscopic cholecystectomy. Br J Surg 2010;97(7):1007-12.

18. Nicholson ML, Kaushik M, Lewis GR, et al. Randomized clinical trial of laparoscopic versus open donor nephrectomy. Br J Surg 2010;97(1):21-8.

19. Tsimogiannis K, Pappas-Gogos G, Benetatos N, et al. Laparoscopic Nissen fundoplication combined with posterior gastropexy in surgical treatment of GERD. Surg Endosc 2010;24(6):1303-9.

20. Degiuli M, Sasako M, Ponti A. Morbidity and mortality in the Italian Gastric Cancer Study Group randomized clinical trial of D1 versus D2 resection for gastric cancer. Br J Surg 2010;97(5):643-9.

21. Liu XX, Jiang ZW, Wang ZM, et al. Multimodal optimization of surgical care shows beneficial outcome in gastrectomy surgery. JPEN J Parenter Enteral Nutr 2010;34(3):313-21.

22. Wang D, KongY, Zhong B, et al. Fast-track surgery improves postoperative recovery in patients with gastric cancer: A randomized comparison with conventional postoperative care. J Gastrointest Surg 2010;14(4):620-7.

23. Rougier P, Sakamoto J, Sargent D, et al. Benefit of adjuvant chemotherapy for resectable gastric cancer: A meta-analysis. JAMA 2010;303(17):1729-37.

24. Jeurnick SM, Polinder S, Steyerberg EW, et al. Cost comparison of gastrojejunostomy versus duodenal stent placement for malignant gastric outlet obstruction. J Gastroenter 2010;45(5):537-43.

25. Villatoro E, Mulla M, Larvin M. Antibiotic therapy for prophylaxis against infection of pancreatic necrosis in acute pancreatitis. Cochrane Database Syst Rev 2010;12(5):CD002941.

26. van Santvoort HC, Besselink MG, Bakker OJ, et al. A step-up approach or open necrosectomy for necrotizing pancreatitis. N Engl J Med 2010;362(16):1491-502.

27. Yang C, Guanghua F, Wei Z, et al. Combination of hemofiltration and peritoneal dialysis in the treatment of severe acute pancreatitis. Pancreas 2010;39(1):16-9.

28. Rogers SJ, Cello JP, Hoen JK, et al. Prospective randomized trial of LC+LCBDE vs ERCP/S+LC for common bile duct stone disease. Arch Surg 2010;145(1):28-33.

29. Zhang W, Xu G, Wu G, et al. Laparoscopic exploration of common bile duct with primary closure versus T-tube drainage: A randomized clinical trial. J Surg Res 2009;157(1):e1-5.

30. Darai E, Dubernard G, Couant C, et al. Randomized trial of laparoscopically assisted versus open colorectal surgery for endometriosis: Morbidity, symptoms, quality of life and fertility. Ann Surg 2010;251(6):1018-23.

31. Swenson BR, Gottschalk A, Wells LT, et al. Intravenous lidocaine is effective as epidural bupivacaine in reducing ileus duration, hospital stay, and pain after open colon resection: A randomized clinical trial. Reg Anesth Pain Med 2010;35(4):370-6.

32. Farid M, Fikry A, El Nakeeb A, et al. Clinical impacts of oral gastrografin follow-through in adhesive small bowel obstruction (SBO). J Surg Res 2010;162(2):170-6.

33. Atkin WS, Edwards R, Kralj-Hans I, et al. Once-only flexible sigmoidoscopy screening in prevention of colorectal cancer: A multicentre randomised controlled trial. Lancet 2010;375(9726):1624-33.

34. Nelson R. Operative procedures for fissure in ano. Cochrane Database Syst Rev 2005;20(1):CD002199.

35. Othman I. Bilateral versus posterior injection of botulinum toxin in the internal anal sphincter for the treatment of acute anal fissure. S Afr J Surg 2010;48(1):20-2.

36. Testini M, Lissidini G, Poli E, et al. A single randomized trial comparing sutures, N-butyl-2-cyanoacrylate and human fibrin glue for mesh fixation during primary inguinal hernia repair. Can J Surg 2010;53(3):155-60.

37. Chlebowski RT, AndersonGL, Gass M, et al. Estrogen and progestin and breast cancer incidence and mortality in postmenopausal women. JAMA 2010;304(15):1684-92.

Index

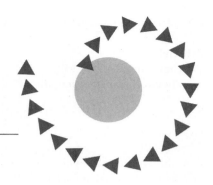

A

Abdominal
  compartment syndrome 113
  procedures 127
  surgery 110
Adjuvant chemotherapy 215
Altemeier's rectosigmoidectomy 128
Aneurysm screening 190
Anorectal discomfort 130
Autonomic neuropathy 3
Axilla in breast cancer 168
Axillary
  lymph node 168
    dissection 173
    node sampling 174

B

Benign peptic stricture 53
Biopsy 209
Brachytherapy 164
Breast 238
  cancer 168

C

Cardiovascular
  diseases 3
  morbidity and mortality 3
Cerebro-vascular disease 3
Chemoradiation therapy 66
Chemotherapy 214
Choice of surgical procedure 126, 131
Chronic
  kidney disease 3
  pancreatitis 53

Colorectal
  cancer 236
  liver metastases 77
Complications of abdominal surgery 110
Conservative methods 143
Consideration of extra hepatic bile duct excision 63
Contrast enhanced CT scan of abdomen 59
Coronary heart disease 3
Cortisol 5
Crohn's disease 109

D

Da Vinci surgical system 228, 239
Dealing with fistula 119
Delorme's procedure 128
Diabetes mellitus 3, 4
Diabetic ketoacidosis 4, 6
Dipeptidyl peptidase-4 16
Disease of axilla 168
Doppler guided haemorrhoidal artery ligation 145
Duodenal stents 51

E

Electrocardiogram 5
Electrolyte balance 6
Endovascular aneurysm repair 183
Enterocutaneous fistula 109
  repair 122
Epinephrine 5
Excision haemorrhoidectomy 145

Extended regional lymphadenectomy 63

External
    beam radiotherapy 159
    pelvic rectal suspension 134

F

Fissure in ano 237
Fistula 110
Fluorine-18-fluorodeoxyglucose 208
Full-thickness rectal prolapse 125

G

Gastric
    carcinoma 230
    outlet obstruction in adults 47
Gastro-oesophageal reflux disease 230
Glucagon like peptide-1 16
Glucocorticoid therapy 12
Glucose insulin potassium infusion 10
Glycaemia 3
GOO caused by malignancy 48
Growth hormone 5

H

Haemorrhoidal artery ligation 145
Haemorrhoids 147
Hand-assisted laparoscopic surgery 228, 229
Hepatocellular carcinoma 74, 81
Hernia 238
Home-made wound vacuum dressing system 224
Hospital volume and upper GI cancer surgery 88
Human epidermal growth factor receptor 2 160
Hyperalimentation 13
Hyperglycaemia 6
Hyperosmolar hyperglycaemic state 6
Hypertension 3
Hypofractionated radiotherapy regimens 160
Hypoglycaemia 4, 6, 12

I

Inflammatory bowel disease 110
Insulin infusions 11

Intensity modulated radiotherapy 161
Internal
    Delorme's procedure 131
    rectal prolapse 129
Intraoperative radiotherapy 162
Ischaemic bowel 113

K

Ketoacidosis 6
Ketosis 5

L

Laparoscopic
    liver resection 73-75
    Nissen fundoplication 230, 239
    sacrocolporectopexy 131
    surgery 228
Length of stay 90
Liver surgery 72
Locally recurrent tumours 215
Loperamide and codeine phosphate 116

M

Magnetic resonance
    angiography 59
    cholangiography 59
Malignant disease 77
Management of
    axilla in breast 168
    GBC 64
    GOO 48
    retroperitoneal sarcoma 205
Metabolic disturbance 47
Metformin therapy 11
Mini-laparoscopic cholecystectomy 229
Modern
    management of intestinal fistula 109
    surgical management of haemorrhoids 141
Monitoring fluid and electrolyte status 117
Myocardial ischaemia 3

N

Neoadjuvant chemotherapy 214

Nonsteroidal anti-inflammatory drugs 225
Nutrition 115, 117

O

Obesity 3
Occasional fresh rectal bleeding 130
Occurrence of fistula 113
Octreotide 116
Open liver resection 74

P

Palliation of jaundice 65
Palliative
    chemotherapy 215
    surgery in advanced gallbladder
        cancer 65
Pancreatic surgery 232
Partial breast radiotherapy 162
Pelvic organ prolapse 136
Perineal procedures 128
Poorly managed surgical catastrophe
    112
Positron emission tomography 59, 208
Posterior rectopexy 127
Post-mastectomy radiotherapy 161
Prevention of GOO 50
Prognostic value of SLNB 170
Proton pump inhibition 47, 116

Q

Quality
    improvement strategies 99
    of surgery 89, 92

R

Radiological staging of axilla 171
Radiotherapy for breast surgeon 159
Reconstructing abdominal wall 120
Rectal and pelvic prolapse 125
Removal of SLNS 170
Resectional rectopexy 127
Retrocolic anastomosis 49
Retroperitoneal sarcomas 205
Rubber band ligation 144

S

Sentinel lymph node biopsy 168
Sepsis 114
Silent myocardial ischaemia 3
Single incision laparoscopic cholecys-
    tectomy 229
Stapled
    haemorrhoidopexy 147
    transanal rectal resection 129, 133
Strategy of surgery 119
Subcutaneous bolus insulin doses 12
Submucosal sclerosant injection 144
Sulfonylurea therapy 11
Surgery for advanced gallbladder
    cancer 57
Surgical
    haemorrhoidectomy 150
    management in advanced cancer 60
    palliation for bowel obstruction 65

T

T3 tumours 61, 63
Therapeutic management of axilla 173
Thiazolidinediones 11
Total parenteral nutrition 13
Transanal haemorrhoidal dearterialisa-
    tion 145
Transversus abdominis plane 225, 239
Treatment of axillary disease 175

U

Unresectable and metastatic disease
    216
Upper GI/HPB 59
Use of biological mesh 121

V

Ventral rectopexy 128

W

Whole breast radiotherapy 159
Wilson's criteria 236